Hospice Care
and Cultural Diversity

Hospice Care
and Cultural Diversity

Donna Lind Infeld, PhD
Audrey K. Gordon, PhD
Bernice Catherine Harper, MSW, MScPH, LLD
Editors

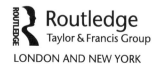

Routledge
Taylor & Francis Group
LONDON AND NEW YORK

First published 1995 by The Haworth Press, Inc.

Published 2013 by Routledge
711 Third Avenue, New York, NY 10017, USA
2 Park Square, Milton Park, Abingdon, Oxfordshire OX14 4RN

First issued in paperback 2016

Routledge is an imprint of the Taylor & Francis Group, an informa business

Hospice Care and Cultural Diversity has also been published as *The Hospice Journal*, Volume 10, Number 2 1995.

Library of Congress Cataloging-in-Publication Data

Hospice care and cultural diversity / Donna Lind Infeld, Audrey K. Gordon, Bernice Catherine Harper, editors.

    p. cm.

includes bibliographical references and index.

ISBN 1-56024-766-5 (alk. paper)

1. Minorities–Hospice care–United States. I. Infeld, Donna Lind. II. Gordon, Audrey K. III. Harper, Bernice Catherine.

R726.8.H655 1995   95-38319

362.1'75–dc20   CIP

ISBN 13: 978-1-138-97199-8 (pbk)

ISBN 13: 978-1-56024-766-1 (hbk)

Hospice Care
and Cultural Diversity

CONTENTS

ABOUT THE EDITORS

Donna Lind Infeld, PhD, is Professor of Health Services Management and Policy and of Health Care Sciences at The George Washington University in Washington, D.C. She is involved in the professional community as Chair of the Association of University Programs in Health Administration Long-Term Care Project Advisory Committees, through elected positions in The Gerontological Society of America, and through membership on the District of Columbia Board of Examiners for Nursing Home Administrators. Dr. Infeld has published numerous long-term care and hospice research articles and co-edited 3 books. She teaches courses in gerontology and long-term care administration, program evaluation, research methods, health information systems, human behavior, and human resources.

Audrey K. Gordon, PhD, is Assistant Professor and Senior Researcher at the University of Illinois School of Public Health. Once President of the Illinois State Hospice Organization, she played a key role in the founding and growth of 4 hospices in the Chicago area. She co-authored *They Need to Know: How to Teach Children About Death*, one of the first books about death education for children. In 1993, Dr. Gordon received the Award of Merit from Northwestern University for her work in thanatology and hospice. She is affiliated with the Professional Advisory Board of Rainbow Hospice, Inc., and a consultant to Unity Hospice, a hospice which specializes in the care of racially and ethnically diverse populations.

Bernice Catherine Harper, MSW, MScPH, LLD, is Medical Care Advisor in the Office of Professional and Business Affairs, Health Care Financing Administration of the Department of Health and Human Services in Washington, D.C. She is Chair of the National Hospice Organization's (NHO) Task Force on Access to Hospice Care by Minority Groups and a member of the Board of Governors of the NHO. Dr. Harper is author of the award-winning book, *Death: The Coping Mechanism of the Health Care Professional*. She was the NHO's 1993 Person-of-the-Year.

Preface

The production of this volume has been an interesting task. The challenges were to identify who was implementing organizational programs of cultural sensitivity and to describe the complex issues arising when working with someone whose culture is different from our own. Barbara Noggle's and Bernice Harper's articles meet the first criterion for organizational implementation and Linda Prong's, Melissa Talamantes' and Michael Beechem's articles, the second. Audrey Gordon's article is adapted from her original research on the health care patterns of Blacks and Hispanics pertaining to hospice access, the hospice organization, and its "user friendliness" to these groups. Patricia Turner-Weeden and Fay A. Burrs provide insight into attitudes toward health care and death in two specific cultures: Native Americans and African Americans, respectively.

One of the things we learned was that many people are *individually knowledgeable and culturally sensitive* but few hospices have systematically planned for service to culturally diverse groups. Over the past two years, one of the editors (AKG) has had the opportunity to work with Unity Hospice in Chicago, which has systematically planned its service to culturally diverse groups in the Chicago metropolitan area. This has been a rewarding and enlightening experience to see Unity Hospice shape communication and service patterns to unique patient needs and cultural family dynamics. Other hospices in the U.S. and Canada are successfully serving such culturally diverse groups as First Americans, Mexican-Americans, Asians, and French-speaking Nova Scotians.

We were especially taken with the comment of a hospice in Hawaii which reported having no minorities! They were *all* different from one another. It would be nice if everyone could say that. Over the course of the past three years, the editors of this volume have grown increasingly uneasy with the word "minority," as it has a pejorative ring. Throughout

[Haworth co-indexing entry note]: "Preface." Gordon, Audrey K. and Bernice Catherine Harper. Co-published simultaneously in *The Hospice Journal* (The Haworth Press, Inc.) Vol. 10, No. 2, 1995, pp. xiii-xiv; and: *Hospice Care and Cultural Diversity* (ed: Donna Lind Infeld, Audrey K. Gordon, and Bernice Catherine Harper) The Haworth Press, Inc., 1995, pp. xiii-xiv. Single or multiple copies of this article are available from The Haworth Document Delivery Service: [1-800-342-9678, 9:00 a.m. - 5:00 p.m. (EST)].

xiii

this volume, various terms are used (Persons of Color, minorities, ethnic groups) as preferred by each author. Overall, we hope the volume begins to capture the richness and some of the differences making up the rich diversity of our country and our American culture.

We learned something else, as well, from putting together this volume. People from many different cultures are eager to share their customs, practices, and beliefs. They want hospice providers to understand their culture and they want their community served by hospice. No one said, "We are the only ones who can take care of our own." Rather, we heard, "We would feel more comfortable if there are people like us in the hospice." This volume then is only a modest effort to acknowledge the efforts of many individuals who work to make hospice comfortably accessible to everyone. We did not identify everyone who is doing this work, nor is our selection of articles inclusive. We hope to encourage research in hospices which are supporting culturally innovative programs–we suspect there is much more going on than is reflected here.

Audrey K. Gordon
Bernice Catherine Harper

Report from the National Task Force on Access to Hospice Care by Minority Groups

Bernice Catherine Harper

SUMMARY. The NHO National Task Force on Access to Hospice Care by Minority Groups, formed in 1987, has undertaken a wide range of activities. In addition to reviewing the research literature, this report summarizes ongoing activities, future goals, and recommended actions for NHO and hospice programs. *[Single or multiple copies of this article are available from The Haworth Document Delivery Service: 1-800-342-9678, 9:00 a.m. - 5:00 p.m. (EST).]*

BACKGROUND

This volume is one result of the dynamic stance taken by the 1987 Board of Directors of the National Hospice Organization (NHO) to

Bernice Catherine Harper, MSW, MScPH, LLD, is Medical Care Advisor, Health Care Financing Administration, Department of Health and Human Services and is Chair of the NHO Task Force on Access to Hospice Care by Minority Groups.

Address correspondence to: Bernice Catherine Harper, MSW, Health Care Financing Administration, Department of Health and Human Services, 200 Independence Avenue, S.W., Washington, D.C. 20201.

The members of the Task Force appreciate the support from the Board of Directors and the Chairperson and Board Liaison, Samira Beckwith; President, John J. Mahoney; and Ole Amundsen, Staff Liaison.

[Haworth co-indexing entry note]: "Report from the National Task Force on Access to Hospice Care by Minority Groups." Harper, Bernice Catherine. Co-published simultaneously in *The Hospice Journal* (The Haworth Press, Inc.) Vol. 10, No. 2, 1995, pp. 1-9; and: *Hospice Care and Cultural Diversity* (ed: Donna Lind Infeld, Audrey K. Gordon, and Bernice Catherine Harper) The Haworth Press, Inc., 1995, pp. 1-9. Single or multiple copies of this article are available from The Haworth Document Delivery Service: [1-800-342-9678, 9:00 a.m. - 5:00 p.m. (EST)].

address a major unmet need in the area of access to hospice care by minority groups. At the request of NHO President, John Mahoney, the NHO Board of Directors established a Task Force on Access to Hospice Care by Minority Groups in August, 1987. Its mandate was to review what, if any, obstacles prevent People of Color[1] from receiving hospice care. The Task Force was further charged to recommend how NHO and local hospice programs could address these issues.

Initial Task Force membership was drawn from the Washington, D.C., metropolitan area and represented a cross-section of People of Color including African Americans, Asians, Native Americans, and Hispanics. In addition providers participated in Task Force activities as a result of news announcements and discussions at the 1987 NHO annual meeting. Although these providers were not appointed to the Task Force, they provided valuable insight about access to hospice care by People of Color.

While recognizing that characteristics other than race determine minority classification (e.g., ethnicity), the Task Force focused on People of Color because a broad exploration of all minority issues was beyond its mandate, scope, and resources. A review of available literature did not reveal any significant national studies about access to hospice care to non-white groups. The most significant hospice research was The National Hospice Study (NHS), conducted by Brown University (Mor et al., 1988). This examination of 26 demonstration sites in the United States compared the cost and quality of hospice care to that received by similar patients in conventional care settings. While not providing patient racial or ethnic characteristics, it did describe the racial makeup of primary caregivers and volunteers. According to the NHS, 8.1 percent of primary caregivers in home health agency-based hospices were non-white, as were 5.3 percent in hospital-based hospices, and 2.7 percent of all hospice volunteers.

An earlier study examined differential patterns of care provided to white and non-white patients. Data on 360 patients cared for over four years at a single hospice was examined. Findings suggested that, on average, white patients received more nursing care time than non-white hospice patients (Burns and Carney, 1984). While the study does not address the question of differential access, it does give some insight into the care provided to People of Color admitted to a hospice program.

Another study reviewed by the Task Force reported on the distribution by sex, race, and age of the hospice patient population in Illinois (Gordon, 1986). Based on responses from approximately 85 percent of the state's hospices, whites accounted for 93.2 percent of patients receiving services during the survey years, 1983-1985. The report noted that many hospices did not maintain records on patient race.

Another study, conducted by the NHO in 1986, examined geographical access to hospice care, defined as being within 25 miles of a hospice program. Almost 95 percent of the population had such geographical access. Exceptions were found in the rural south and west. For example, Mississippi and North Dakota had limited access with only 48.5 percent and 59.7 percent of the population, respectively, living within 25 miles of a hospice program.

After review of the literature, the Task Force concluded that there was inadequate data about access to hospice care by People of Color. As a preliminary data-gathering step, each member and other contacts completed a brief questionnaire about perceived barriers to minority access to hospice programs.

Based on these findings and the literature review, the Task Force concluded that hospice care was not readily available and/or utilized by People of Color. With notable exceptions, it appeared that hospices had been unsuccessful in serving non-white communities proportionally to their presence in the potential hospice population. The Task Force further concluded that this lack of utilization was due, in part, to the absence of targeted information for consumers and health professionals about hospice care in the non-white community. This may be caused by low priority given to marketing hospice services to the community at large. Another reason for lack of access to hospice care for non-white populations was their lack of financial resources for access to medical care in general. Hospice care may be viewed as a luxury compared with other pressing economic and health needs of many non-white patients and their families. Finally, cultural differences on issues related to death and dying may not be understood by hospices founded and staffed predominantly by members of the white middle class.

In 1988, the Task Force made the following recommendations to the NHO Board of Directors about how NHO can assist with promoting minority access to hospice care:

1. Increase statistical monitoring of ethnic and racial characteristics of staff and board members and of patients.
2. Encourage staff, board, and committee education.
3. Continue liaison with national organizations representing People of Color.
4. Encourage local hospice to become culturally sensitive and culturally diverse.
5. Create an Advisory Council on Minority Affairs.
6. Address special cultural needs of patients with AIDS.
7. Continue recruitment of the Task Force.

Based on these recommendations a new format for workshops on cultural issues was adopted for NHO Annual meetings. Cultural values and beliefs are now presented by individuals representing various cultural groups.

ONGOING ACTIVITIES OF THE NATIONAL TASK FORCE

According to Ann MacGregor, former Chair of the NHO, "Something is going on in the heartland regarding People of Color."[2] Progress has been made in increasing awareness about access to hospice care by minorities. The significant role of the Task Force, reaching a national membership of 30 providers from 14 states and the District of Columbia, received some of the credit. Presentations of the National Task Force include the following:

1. Workshops and seminars on cultural diversity and grief at each Annual NHO meeting.
2. In 1990, the Task Force sponsored a national conference, "Meeting the Needs of Terminally Ill Persons of Color and Their Families." This conference introduced hospice care to the leadership of national organizations representing culturally diverse groups. It demonstrated the value of hospice care in improving quality of life. Louis W. Sullivan, M.D., then Secretary of the Department of Health and Human Services, was the keynote speaker. His speech, "Minority Health and Hospice Care," was published by the NHO and 2,000 copies were distributed to hospices and other health care providers.
3. Task Force members participated in a successful Regional Conference in Boston, Massachusetts, in 1991, at the J.F. Kennedy Library. This invitational educational conference, "Improving Access to Hospice Care for People of Color," was co-sponsored by Trinity Hospice, Boston, Massachusetts; Home Health and Hospice Care of Nashua, New Hampshire; Heritage Home Health of Meredith, New Hampshire; and the National Hospice Organization.
4. Presentations about hospice care were made at Town Hall Meetings in local minority churches and/or at the Symposium hotel during NHO annual meetings in Detroit (1990), Seattle (1991), Nashville, (1992), Salt Lake City (1993), and Washington, D.C. (1994). These meetings involved local leaders, religious institutions, and other health care and social care organizations.
5. The National Hospice Organization's *Resolution on Access to Hospice Care* was approved by the membership in 1992 (See Appendix).

6. Task Force members participated in eight programs including local, state, and national conferences about access to hospice care for minorities.

In addition to these presentations, the Task Force also staffed a booth and distributed information at NHO meetings and to other organizations and programs about minority access, minority hiring, and appointing minority board members.

The Task Force was an active presence at the NHO's Sixteenth Annual Symposium and Exposition in October, 1994, in Washington, D.C. The conference theme, "Opening Doors: The Next Generation of Hospice Caring," echoed the access theme the Task Force represents. There was much excitement at the Task Force's booth in the exposition hall, where the handbook, *Caring for Our Own: The Hospice Way,* was distributed to hospice representatives from across the nation. This NHO publication contains models of activities, concrete actions, and resources to be used by hospices in their quest to provide appropriate and culturally sensitive hospice care to people of color, children, the disadvantaged, the underserved, and persons with AIDS. The Handbook supports NHO's goal of providing universal access to hospice care for all terminally ill individuals and their families. Task Force members Virginia Swaggard, Charletta Marshall, and Thaiti Weaver served as Chair and Co-Chairs of the booth, respectively.

The Task Force also sponsored its fifth Annual Town Hall Meeting on serving People of Color. Presentations included dynamic cultural frames of reference in death and dying presented by Sydney Billingsley, Bernadine C. Dailey, Grace Lee, Dr. J.T. Garrett, and Samira K. Beckwith. Jeffrey Munks, Director of Marketing for AT&T Language Line Services, gave a living testimony on "Crossing the Language Barriers" through the use of the AT&T Language Line, currently available for 160 languages. A demonstration on the importance of language, cultural patterns and behavior relative to hospice caregivers and service providers was given by Dr. Rodewell Catoe, former Deputy Chief of Police, District of Columbia, and more recently, a professor of human development at the University of Maryland.

Dr. Bernice Catherine Harper participated in a flag raising ceremony at the Model Cities Senior Wellness Center in northeast Washington. The new flag designed exclusively for the NHO was unveiled for the first time at this event. The NHO donated a new flag pole to the Center in appreciation of their support of hospice care. "The raising of the hospice flag symbolizes the remarkable growth of the hospice movement since its inception two decades ago and serves to remind us that hospice care must be delivered wherever it is needed, whenever it is needed, and in whatever language is needed to make it understandable" (Dr. Bernice Catherine Harper, 1994).

The National Task Force has also identified hospice programs which have successful minority outreach programs, provided technical assistance and consultation to hospices trying to increase access to minority groups, networked with state organizations, and published articles in *Hospice* and *Newsline*. This publication is one of the crowning accomplishments of Task Force activities.

FUTURE GOALS FOR THE TASK FORCE

At its March 1992 meeting, NHO President John Mahoney emphasized that the Task Force's goal is to change the hospice community in general, not just the NHO. Although the number of minority patients served by hospice had increased in the last five years from 5 to 8 percent, those numbers still fall far short. With this in mind, the Task Force set the following agenda:

Expansion of Services

In order for hospices to successfully expand their services into minority communities, they must establish a pattern of education and communication appropriate to both white and non-white consumers and professionals. Consumers can be targeted through churches, service organizations, schools, and health care programs. Health care professionals can be reached through professional societies, hospitals, clinics, and social service agencies.

Communication and education must be presented in positive terms. They should be framed with the understanding that clinical services delivered outside the hospital may be perceived by People of Color to be of poorer quality. Hospice philosophy may be seen as giving up on trying to stay alive and, as in many cultures, in conflict with the wishes and prayers of the patient's family and supporters.

Everyone needs information on hospice before the crisis of an impending death reaches them. Professionals need to be able to explain the hospice concept with sensitivity to the cultural background of the family needing help. Hospices must be able to accommodate, through staffing and practice, the cultural differences of various communities, and staff must be educated about diverse attitudes toward death and dying.

To be successful, hospices must be aware of the significant role churches and clergy play in minority communities. Hospice leaders must work collaboratively with churches which can also be an excellent forum for educating and recruiting volunteers. Using volunteers with ties to the minority community is critical to promoting community knowledge about hospices and acceptance of the hospice concept of care. Educational materials used to promote hospices must reflect ethnic and cultural differences. Hospice programs need to recruit and place members of the minority community in positions of leadership both on the staff and on boards of directors.

How the NHO Can Help

- The NHO, as well as individual hospices, should continue monitoring the ethnic and racial background of hospice staff and of patients/families who receive services.
- The NHO should continue offering educational programs to educate and sensitize hospice professionals about the needs of minority groups. These programs should be based on the recognition that significant differences exist among minority groups in practices and attitudes about death and dying. The entry point for access to hospice care may also be different for each group.
- Educational programs must also be provided on a regional basis, using local faculty and a standard curriculum. Programs on ethnicity, culture, and access to hospice care by People of Color should be continued as part of the Annual Meeting and Symposium and should also be addressed in a plenary session.
- People of Color involved in hospice roles should be part of the outreach and teaching staff for NHO programs and be involved in developing a curricula about the groups they represent.
- The NHO should maintain current reference materials about the cultural meaning of death and dying in non-white communities.
- The NHO should continue sponsoring programs to establish liaisons with national organizations representing People of Color, to foster the concept of hospice care for non-white groups, and consult on hospices to these groups. State hospice organizations should also be encouraged to do the same at the state level.
- The NHO should continue to address the needs of minority populations for hospice care. The Task Force should have access to the NHO board of directors to assure continued cultural and ethnic sensitivity. NHO Services and publications must reflect sensitivity to the issues of People of Color and provide models for state and local organizations to use in developing their own programs, projects, task forces, and other mechanisms.

What Hospices Can Do

- Hospice programs should be encouraged to review their service patterns to see if they are adequately reaching all residents of their service area. If they are not, they should contact local minority leaders to see how their communities can participate in hospices. Hospices should provide community education and targeted marketing.
- The status and involvement of volunteers in the communities of People of Color are unknown. While there remains a need to recruit non-white volunteers to serve in hospices, it is also critical to recruit People of Color to hospice staff positions and to state, local, and national board membership.

AIDS AND PEOPLE OF COLOR

The fastest growing sub-groups of people who have tested sero-positive for HIV are People of Color. The NHO, through its AIDS Resource Committee, must continue its activities on behalf of People of Color who have AIDS. This population must be considered in any policy and any additional technical assistance the NHO develops.

The National Task Force on Access to Hospice Care by Minority Groups applauds the initiative taken by the NHO Board. In a time of mergers, consolidations, and emphasis on cost cutting and profit making, it is encouraging to see a national health association provide leadership in seeking to expand services to underserved groups.

NOTES

1. For purposes of this report the Task Force uses the phrases People of Color and non-white interchangeably to define those individuals who would be considered minorities by race.

2. Note to Bernice Catherine Harper, March 8, 1991.

REFERENCES

Burns, N., and Carney, N. (1984). Patterns of hospice care: The RN Role. *The Hospice Journal, 2*(1).

Gordon, (1986). Survey for the Illinois Hospice Organization. Unpublished data.

Mor, V., Greer, D.S., Kastenbaum, R. (Eds.) (1988). *The Hospice Experiment.* Baltimore: The Johns Hopkins Press.

APPENDIX

NATIONAL HOSPICE ORGANIZATION'S
RESOLUTION ON ACCESS TO HOSPICE CARE

WHEREAS, The National Hospice Organization is considered the voice of the Nation's hospice community; and,

WHEREAS, The members of the National Hospice Organization support the principle of access to hospice care for all terminally ill individuals regardless of age, gender, nationality, race, creed, sexual orientation, disability, diagnosis, availability of primary caregiver, or ability to pay; and,

WHEREAS, The members of the National Hospice Organization support the sharing of information and experience on creative ways to remove barriers to such access; and,

WHEREAS, The National Hospice Organization is a national leader in the provision of education, networking opportunities, technical assistance and public policy advocacy; therefore,

RESOLVED, That the National Hospice Organization rededicate its efforts to reach the goal of universal access to hospice care for terminally ill individuals in the United States.

Approved by the NHO Membership on May 5, 1992.

EDITORIAL ESSAYS

Death and Dying
from a Native American Perspective

Patricia Turner-Weeden

We, as Native Americans, view this earthly plain as a world of learning experiences. Creator has placed us here for a little while. Some view it as a journey. We have come with many gifts from Creator; and these gifts are meant to be shared. Along with our gifts, we have been given instructions by the Great One, who knows all and sees all; for this we are thankful.

Because we are here for a little while, it is most important that we attempt to carry out Creator's teachings. All things are to be learned. The tests are difficult; once learned never forgotten.

As we journey around the sacred hoop of life, at the point of the four directions, we learn lessons. Some journey at a rapid rate, others slower, knowing we don't wish to hasten our time here before we journey on to the other world.

Patricia Turner-Weeden is a Nurse/Educator at the North American Indian Center of Boston, Inc.

Address correspondence to: Patricia Turner-Weeden, North American Indian Center of Boston, Inc., 105 South Huntington Avenue, Jamaica Plain, MA 02130.

[Haworth co-indexing entry note]: "Death and Dying from a Native American Perspective." Turner-Weeden, Patricia. Co-published simultaneously in *The Hospice Journal* (The Haworth Press, Inc.) Vol. 10, No. 2, 1995, pp. 11-13; and: *Hospice Care and Cultural Diversity* (ed: Donna Lind Infeld, Audrey K. Gordon, and Bernice Catherine Harper) The Haworth Press, Inc., 1995, pp. 11-13. Single or multiple copies of this article are available from The Haworth Document Delivery Service: [1-800-342-9678, 9:00 a.m. - 5:00 p.m. (EST)].

11

Our Native Peoples believe we pass-over into the spirit world, where we are met by our ancestors who have passed on before us. This world is a world of love and beauty, not to be feared. Many who have had a near death experience state it was a difficult choice to make, whether to remain in the spirit world or to journey back to this earthly plain. Some have chosen to return to their human forms, others wish to remain in the spiritual state of being. We, as Native Americans, believe our spirits live on. Our outer shells deteriorate, but our spirits choose this outer covering or vessel while we are here on our journey.

I personally believe in reincarnation. When I say this, I am not speaking for all Native Americans. I feel I have journeyed through here many times. I fear no death; I feel we will all meet again at another time and place as Creator continues to cross our paths with others.

When our time arrives to meet our Makers, many have fear and doubt. They know what this world is like but they don't know what the other world is like. They don't trust the Great One that placed them here initially. We, as human beings, tend to fear the unknown—and later realize our fears were unfounded.

I have worked as a Hospice Nurse many times. In some of my cases, I have seen clients and their families not willing to let go of each other and material things. We cannot hold on to the past; the past will take care of itself. Native people have been instructed not to hold onto materialistic things; to do so is known in our way as greed. Mother always said, "You came into the world with nothing and you will go out with nothing."

As we prepare to pass-over, I firmly believe our Creator lets us know our work here on earth is coming to an end. We must relinquish our task and make way for new growth and ideas.

One day I met a young man and his family. We had not seen each other in a long time. We inquired about each other's family. I shared how my oldest son had recently passed-over. The young man was like a brother to my son; they had played together while growing up. The young man started to cry, he too had lost a loved one, his grandfather. He made a statement, "I learned so much from my grandfather. He had so much knowledge in his head, and now it's gone." He felt sad about this. Later I shared this with a Medicine Man I had met. He said, "This young man was greedy for the knowledge his grandfather had. Grandfather had given all he could while here." We should not want for more, we must be thankful for what we receive from our elders. We must not hold onto them in this way. Trying to hold on is disturbing to both parties. Frustration is felt on both sides, the one preparing to pass-over and the individual or families which remain.

This should be a time of peace and understanding–a time to communicate, if at all possible; to settle differences, to make peace with ourselves and others. Then we are prepared to take the next step through the "Big Open Door" into the spirit world, to greet our Creator and all of our ancestors.

Many times we can validate this to be a true experience. We hear those preparing to leave describing visits from their husband, wife, mother, father, or others who have passed-over. The visitors come to assist them or help them make a smooth transition over to the other side.

We must remember never to hasten this experience by taking our own lives. We must view our bodies as temples, gifts from Creator; to be cared for in the best way possible. Creator has placed us here, it is up to him to determine when we must leave.

I have shared this essay with many of my clients. They have found peace and contentment in their final days. They have learned to let go, and go in peace.

May Creator nurture us spiritually and in all ways, to make this a beautiful and enlightening experience.

To this I say Ho.

The African American Experience: Breaking the Barriers to Hospices

Fay A. Burrs

SUMMARY. The lack of understanding of the historical perspectives and cultural factors impact all aspects of hospice care for African Americans. This article addresses these areas in a broad context as well as the skills, behavior, and performance required to provide appropriate, competent, and culturally sensitive care to the terminally ill and dying African American and other culturally diverse population groups. *[Single or multiple copies of this article are available from The Haworth Document Delivery Service: 1-800-342-9678, 9:00 a.m. - 5:00 p.m. (EST).]*

INTRODUCTION

People of Color are growing in number and are increasingly becoming consumers of hospice services. What barriers prevent them from accepting this well-intended and desperately needed care? Many health care professionals, both African American and White, believe there is little difference in the way you approach the dynamics of care for African Americans. This may arise because both are educated from European and American per-

Fay A. Burrs, BSN, RN, is Director of Hospice Home Care/Home Health Services at The Washington Home. She was formerly NHO's Nurse Section Leader for The Council of Hospice Professionals.

Address correspondence to: Fay A. Burrs, RN, Hospice of Washington, 3720 Upton Street, N.W., Washington, D.C. 20016.

[Haworth co-indexing entry note]: "The African American Experience: Breaking the Barriers to Hospices." Burrs, Fay A. Co-published simultaneously in *The Hospice Journal* (The Haworth Press, Inc.) Vol. 10, No. 2, 1995, pp. 15-18; and: *Hospice Care and Cultural Diversity* (ed: Donna Lind Infeld, Audrey K. Gordon, and Bernice Catherine Harper) The Haworth Press, Inc., 1995, pp. 15-18. Single or multiple copies of this article are available from The Haworth Document Delivery Service: [1-800-342-9678, 9:00 a.m. - 5:00 p.m. (EST)].

spectives, believing that most families have the same basic drives, motivations, and psycho-dynamics. I would assert that the assumption that there are no differences forms the basis of barriers to delivering care to African American or other minority families. While we are all Americans, there are differences.

HISTORICAL PERSPECTIVE

These differences stem from our different histories. For African Americans, that history is rooted in slavery; the horrible time when we were forcibly merged with a foreign culture. Almost 400 years ago, our ancestors were stolen or sold from our motherland. They were transported in subhuman conditions, including chains and manacles, and considered property to be sold at the whim of the slave master. Families were separated and women exploited as breeders. Men were forced into powerlessness and subservience. Next came the Civil War, when our people were emancipated into quasi-freedom of second-class citizenship. African American lives were still expendable and of little value. Lynching African American men was public entertainment, efforts continued to keep them in their place. Segregation, prejudice, and unfairness were found from water fountains to public parks.

Brought from Africa was a strong spiritual belief that God is in control of all; that no good thing will be withheld. Throughout our enslavement we continued to trust God. We carry on with the strength of our ancestors to fight for equality and justice in this land we helped build with our backs, our blood, out might. Fight we must and demand we did. Despite beatings and dogs, we began marching to register to vote and make our voices heard. We marched to make known our stand that our freedom and quality was worth dying for . . . and some did. With Black Power, Black Panther, and Black Pride, we began to reclaim the pride of our heritage. We began to fight within the system, through education, law, politics, religion, and family. We are proud to represent many countries . . . to be People of Color . . . and Americans.

IMPACT ON ATTITUDES TOWARD HOSPICE CARE

It is necessary to recount this history to explain why many African Americans have difficulty trusting most health care providers and trusting the system. The goal of retelling this history is to bring you face to face with the experience of African Americans in this country. We can't deny this history or continuing prejudice today. Barriers created by this history to provision of hospice care to African Americans include lack of trust, fear, hopelessness, lack of knowledge, and inability to identify with providers.

Lack of Trust

Throughout history, having been treated as second class citizens, African Americans have frequently received unequal treatment and inadequate medical care. This has created a tradition and culture of distrust.

It is critical not to violate African American patients' developing trust. Promise only what you can deliver and to deliver everything you promise. Broken faith and sunken hope has been too much a part of the African American history. Further, do not presume to "understand" how the patient and family feel. You can say you will "try to understand," but that is very different from claiming to actually understand.

Fear

Fear stems from generations of stories of mysterious disappearances of family members. Fear of experimental or second-class health care, combined with unfamiliarity with the hospice concept leads to resistance and apprehension toward providers.

Hopelessness

Hopelessness has evolved from being denied access to options throughout life. Why should access to terminal treatment be any different? This feeling, combined with the hopelessness of terminal disease itself, can breed depression and despair.

Lack of Knowledge

Even within the Caucasian population, hospice is not well recognized or understood. The African American community doesn't understand hospice and hospice doesn't understand them. This is a major gap to cross.

Inability to Identify with Providers

Very few hospice caregivers or volunteers are African Americans. When providers do not have a common cultural background with patients, the ability to support, nurture, and promote maximum independence is threatened.

OVERCOMING BARRIERS

In order to overcome these barriers, providers need to develop a deeper sensitivity and heightened awareness of the patient's needs, be informed of cultural attitudes and traditions, learn about community resources, and become a therapeutic team player to the patient and family.

As with all patients, it is critical to recognize that each person and family is unique. Their coping mechanisms and defenses are unique. This individuality must be respected, even if it includes denial to the end.

The tradition of honoring and respecting the great spirit of African ancestors leads to discomfort with death in the home. It may take group support, involvement of clergy, and ongoing support to overcome this resistance.

Some of the skills that can help providers overcome barriers among African American families require personal growth on the part of caregivers. We must become sensitive to our own biases, learn to empower our patients and their families, and develop trusting and therapeutic relationships. As organizations we need to identify an appropriate target group to serve, design an fitting strategy to meet their needs, develop relationships throughout the community, and assure accurate information is used as the basis for planning and service delivery.

RESEARCH REPORTS

Maria:
Developing a Culturally-Sensitive
Treatment Plan in Pre-Hospice South Texas

Michael H. Beechem

SUMMARY. This is a case study of a young Mexican-American woman who suffered from end-stage renal disease and severe depression in Texas, before the availability of hospice care. The patient, while struggling to retain her cultural identity in a renal care unit which stressed efficiency, was labeled noncompliant by the medical team. Through knowledge gained from staff discussions, the medical team was able to integrate cultural sensitivity and hospice principles into the treatment plan. With an increased focus on her psychosocial needs, the patient was able to die with a sense of dignity and cultural integrity. *[Single or multiple copies of this article are available from The Haworth Document Delivery Service: 1-800-342-9678, 9:00 a.m. - 5:00 p.m. (EST).]*

Michael H. Beechem, PhD, MSW, is Assistant Professor in the Department of Social Work at The University of West Florida.

Address correspondence to: Michael H. Beechem, PhD, Department of Social Work, The University of West Florida, 11000 University Parkway, Pensacola, FL 32514-5751.

[Haworth co-indexing entry note]: "Maria: Developing a Culturally-Sensitive Treatment Plan in Pre-Hospice South Texas." Beechem, Michael H. Co-published simultaneously in *The Hospice Journal* (The Haworth Press, Inc.) Vol. 10, No. 2, 1995, pp. 19-34; and: *Hospice Care and Cultural Diversity* (ed: Donna Lind Infeld, Audrey K. Gordon, and Bernice Catherine Harper) The Haworth Press, Inc., 1995, pp. 19-34. Single or multiple copies of this article are available from The Haworth Document Delivery Service: [1-800-342-9678, 9:00 a.m. - 5:00 p.m. (EST)].

BACKGROUND

In 1976, as a recently graduated masters-level social worker from the upper midwest, I accepted a position in a South Texas hospital to provide social services to end-stage renal disease patients. While inexperienced in working with dying patients, through my studies I had come to appreciate the value of humane care for dying persons as well as their right to autonomy in decision-making about medical care.

The following account is a case study that required cultural sensitivity and contained elements of hospice philosophy and practice at a time when formalized hospice services were virtually unknown in South Texas. Hospice philosophy and practice in this case study included: caring as opposed to curing; controlling pain; providing emotional support for patients; treating family members and the patient as a unit; involving the patient and family members in care planning; relaxing visitation policies; applying an interdisciplinary team approach; and, above all, regarding the dying person as unique with special needs.

I met Maria Garcia when she began hospital-based dialysis. Unlike many of the patients who blindly resigned themselves to a rigid medical regimen, Maria questioned all facets of the treatment. I was fascinated with her independence and spunk and decided to maintain extensive case notes to better understand this refreshingly free-spirited person; therefore, notes and an unpublished videotaped interview provide much of the material for this case study.

Maria, a twenty-one year old Mexican-American woman, was diagnosed with end-stage renal disease during a routine office visit for acute chest pains. Had Maria lived at home in her small South Texas town, she would have sought a remedy through a cuarandero, a practitioner of rural folk medicine. However, the excruciating pain in her chest was unbearable and she did not know of a local cuarandero. It is not known how long Maria suffered from these chest pains, but, according to Clark (1970), Mexican-Americans will "try to 'be strong' and often refuse to accept the fact they are sick until they become acutely ill" (p. 198). De La Rosa (1989) writes that:

> Age-adjusted data on use of physician visits indicate that Mexican-Americans averaged fewer visits to a physician (3.7) than white and black non-Hispanic Americans (4.8 and 4.7 visits, respectively) and that Puerto Ricans and Cuban Americans averaged more visits (6.0 and 6.2 visits, respectively). (Trevino, 1984, p. 109)

After undergoing dialysis treatment for two months at a Houston clinic, Maria decided to return to her parents, seven sisters, and three brothers in

South Texas. She reasoned that she could receive dialysis in Corpus Christi and benefit from the emotional support of her family who lived 50 miles to the south. Her family had opposed her move to Houston two and a half years before because they felt she should stay with the family in rural Texas, near the Mexican border. Her mother had forewarned her that misfortune could come to her in a big city away from the family.

In a later hospitalization, Maria expressed the concern that she had been punished for leaving her home. As a third generation Mexican-American, her cultural heritage remained very much a part of her. Clark (1970) relates a case study of a Mexican woman who suffered from gastro-intestinal upsets after moving to the United States as punishment for leaving her home for an "artificial environment." Clark writes that illness:

> . . . is a means of dramatizing to others the evil consequences of cultural change and of defending the 'old ways'–Mexican customs and traditions which are under constant attack in the United States. This is done by attributing disease to the demands of Anglo society or to ways of American life which are uncongenial to the patient. (p. 201)

Rosen (1990) writes that "ethnic characteristics are transmitted through the generations and are part of the historical makeup (vertical influence) of the family in the present" (p. 148). Sotomayor (1989) offers a logical explanation of how the cultural heritage is retained by even a third generation Mexican-American when she explains the "Culture of Migration . . . gets renewed and revitalized on an almost daily basis on this side of the border, reaffirming its symbols, values, beliefs and customs to pass on to the next generation" (p. 58).

CASE ASSESSMENT

I was asked to work closely with Maria because the nephrologist reported that "she is a very unmanageable patient and we can ill afford any disruptions. I'm also concerned that she refuses to follow her medications." Strauss and Glaser (1975) suggest that noncompliance of the medical regimen may relate to denial of the disease. They report that "if the patient simply denies that he has the disease, he may refuse to submit to a regimen or may only minimally carry it out" (p. 25). Hyland (1978) suggests that it is common for patients to react to scolding from the medical staff by deliberate noncompliance with medications.

In our first meeting it was apparent that Maria was deeply distressed.

She bitterly criticized virtually every facet of the hospital's operations, from the nurses to the food. "The food, if you want to call it that, is sickening," she stressed. "If I could just have some of Mamma's carne guisada or maybe some chicken mole. Oh God, if I could just return to the good old days, even if just for a few moments," she bemoaned. Parkes (cited in Schneider, 1984) reports a yearning to return to the "good old days" before the loss occurred (p. 132). For Maria, the "good old days" signified a family "fiesta" embellished with Mexican food and music, attended by her parents, brothers and sisters, grandparents, aunts and uncles, and cousins. "How much must one give up to get well? My whole culture?" Maria felt a keen sense of cultural loss from hospital policy preventing Mexican food and music, and her family's cohesiveness was threatened by a rule disallowing visitation by her sister based on age. She also angrily criticized the dialysis nurses whom she described as "uncaring, efficient witches dressed up as nurses. Why they even threatened to make me take dialysis alone in that room, separate from the unit, if I didn't keep quiet."

Maria related a situation that occurred immediately before she dialyzed for the first time. A dialysis nurse asked her how she was doing and Maria began what no doubt developed into a bitterly critical dissertation on the hospital's state of affairs when suddenly a nurse "cut me off and said I'd feel a lot better and get well faster if I'd stop complaining so much. Oh, yes. She also said 'don't worry about a thing, honey. Just sit back and we'll take care of everything.' Can you imagine? My first day of dialysis in this stupid hospital and I'm hooked up to this monster that looks like an umbilical cord!" Rosen (1990) identifies a "Preparatory Phase" (Phase I of anticipatory grieving) in which "the blame is often placed on 'stupid doctors' who have given bad advice or on 'insensitive nurses'" (p. 73). On the other hand, Maria may have been realistic about the nurses' treatment of her.

Maria's autonomy was assaulted by the many hospital rules, the dialysis machine, the emphasis on efficiency and seemingly everything being done for her. She felt emotionally suffocated, helpless, and without control. "Learned helplessness" is often experienced by chronically-ill patients who experience a deep loss of control over their medical decisions. Seligman (1975) warns that depression develops from a sense that one's situation will not change, no matter what action is taken. Kalish (1985) describes the term "learned helplessness" is used to refer to an emotion and related behaviors that occur when people believe there is nothing they can do to avoid punishment or to obtain satisfaction.

Strauss and Glaser (1975) caution that there is an extreme variation between the amount of responsibility the patient assumes at home and that allowed at a hospital. Frequently, the patient assumes "almost total responsibility when . . . at home, and the medical staff will assume most of the responsibility when the patient is hospitalized" (p. 144). Strauss and Glaser (1975) write that staff members can "thereby not only save themselves much trouble with so-called difficult patients but greatly contribute to the betterment of the care" (p. 144) by considering the patients' views in treatment planning.

Clearly, if Maria were to benefit from her care, she would need to participate in the treatment plan, gain some control over decision making, and become empowered regarding choices. These are key issues in the hospice philosophy of care which were not well-known in hospitals at that time. Issues with the nursing staff required attention as well. The nurse had misunderstood Maria's anger; she interpreted Maria's attack as personal, and her recourse was the punitive threat of isolation. Maria had said, "I am depending on the staff for everything and I hate them for this. I sometimes feel that I can't do anything for myself, and I've always been such an independent person." Maria further described the feeling as being "stripped of everything. My personality, my whole self is being stripped. The doctor does this and the technicians and nurses do that for me. My food is delivered to me and I have no choice in selecting it. It's got to the point where I often wonder if I am capable of doing anything for myself." I wasn't clear how she could address these problems since the hospital's authority seemed difficult to challenge or change.

Whenever Maria suffered a relapse and required additional dialysis and medical care, the medical staff provided increased attention; then, when personal interactions with her diminished, she would return to a deeply depressed state. The staff also made an effort to exert greater control over Maria's life, as was evident by limiting visitations by family and friends. In an almost punitive, nagging manner, Maria would be reminded of what would happen should she not follow her strict diet and medications, and that meant absolutely no Mexican food from her mother and sisters. The staff's attitude toward Maria was paternalistic and condescending.

The nephrologist advised Maria about what he would do for her rather than involving her in the planning and decision-making processes. Although Maria would never fully regain the life she had before beginning dialysis, one of my goals was for her to regain some semblance of the autonomy and independence she had before the imposition of a highly stringent, regimented medical plan of care. She desperately needed to exercise some autonomy and control over her life.

Besides hypertension and end-stage renal disease, Maria learned that she was diabetic and that her heart was malfunctioning. The nephrologist informed her that she would need heart surgery if she ever expected to live a normal life. Maria countered with "I am sick and tired of having my body abused. You people stick me every time I'm hooked up to that horrible machine. Three times I've had surgery and it hasn't helped. You refuse to treat me as a whole person with feelings. Now this! No, I will not allow you or anyone else to butcher me anymore. If I die because I refuse another operation, then so be it!" Cassell (1974) reports that in our technologically-oriented society terminally-ill patients are frequently treated as objects and not as people with feelings.

The Cuarandero's Role

On several occasions, Maria had sought the services of a cuarandera, whom she was convinced provided more effective treatment than did the physicians. In Mexican folk medicine a cuarandero is a spiritual leader with healing powers. It is common even in the U.S. for Mexican-Americans to seek out cuaranderos rather than physicians. According to Falicov (cited in McGoldrick, Pearce, & Giordano, 1982),

> The use of folk medicine occasionally surfaces when treating families of Mexican descent who maintain two systems of beliefs and practices regarding illness and health. The most prevalent [sic practice] is modern Western medicine, but some families still practice curanderismo [sic] (rural folk medicine) either before, after or simultaneously with modern remedies. (p. 146-147)

Because treatment is holistic and involves a deep concern for spiritual needs, it is not surprising that cuaranderos can claim a relatively high success rate in the treatment of psychosomatic illnesses. Cuaranderismo, unlike modern Western medicine, stresses the significance of interpersonal relationships.

The cuarandera is perceived by patients as more than a practitioner. According to Clark (1970), "people know that she is one of them and that she really cares what happens to them and has their welfare at heart" (p. 208). She is also a friend who has established a close relationship with the patient. Clark adds that "folk concepts of disease from Mexico are still important to Mexican-Americans; many of the beliefs persist in the thinking of 2nd-3rd generation" (p. 163). McGoldrick et al. (1982) add that "it is interesting that even folk illnesses are often attributed to interpersonal problems such as envy" (p. 147).

Maria's Father

At an earlier point in her treatments, Maria had shown signs of accepting her condition and appeared philosophical about the prospects of dying. Subsequently she lapsed into a depressed state characterized by a profound sense of helplessness which she related in part to feelings about her father. Señor Garcia, a fiercely proud person and the titular head of La Familia, was painfully struggling with denial of Maria's medical problems and impending death. Maria began feeling intense discomfort and guilt about her father's anguish. Rolando Ramirez (1993), a South Texas Veterans Administration social worker with an extensive Mexican-American clientele, asserts that "frequently the female family members will assume responsibility for the male's feelings. Understanding their (the males) needs to appear in charge of situations and to not appear weak, the male family members will not usually be encouraged to express feelings of grief." All of Maria's family members were experiencing emotional pain, but it was her father who suffered most, in spite of his efforts to mask it. Maria often remarked that she wished her father would visit her more often, but she knew that seeing her so sick was too much of an ordeal for him.

According to Clark (1970), the "Patriarchal authoritarian family pattern" is misunderstood by the casual observer, because wives will often give the pretense of subservience and then "openly defy male authority" by assuming major decision-making roles (p. 150). In effect, the males give the pretense of being in charge with respect paid to their male role, but the females are often the ones who are the catalysts in affecting change. Clark (1970) insists that "the change toward a more equal relationship between spouses is not always apparent to Anglo observers, however" (p. 150). Falicov (cited in McGoldrick et al., 1982) writes that "although in most Mexican marriages there is outward compliance with the cultural ideal of male dominance and female submission, this is often a social fiction" (p. 134). Falicov further adds that in their private lives, "Mexican-American females may include husbands who are domineering and patriarchal, who are submissive and dependent on their wives for major decisions, or who follow a more egalitarian power structure" (p. 134). Even though Señor Garcia outwardly portrayed the authoritarian patriarchal leader, he looked to Maria and her mother for emotional strength. Matriarchal dominance has its origin in Mexico where the elderly woman is known as una torre (a tower). Lewis (cited in Cowgill, 1986) describes the activities of an elderly Mexican woman who:

> . . . visited her son's home daily, usually arriving before noon, criticized the daughter-in-law's housekeeping, re-arranged furniture,

supervised grandchildren, berated her son for his infidelity to his
wife, and gave advice liberally. (p. 88)

According to Cowgill (1986), it is common for the elderly female to
assume a dominant role in the household while "the elderly male is more
likely to reach a plateau in activity and esteem" (p. 118).

The sources of Maria's depression were multifaceted: she was deeply
troubled about her father's emotional struggle; she experienced a loss of
control caused mostly from a highly-structured treatment regimen; and she
felt stress associated with the medical staff's lack of empathy toward her
illness. Finally, she felt a loss of a culturally-centered life style.

Intervention Requested

A few months after being assigned to Maria, I received a memo from
the Technical Director expressing alarm at Maria's refusal to follow a
low-sodium diet and her refusal to take her hypertension medication. I
wondered whether her noncompliance was in retaliation to the authority of
the Technical Director–who in a condescending manner constantly reminded Maria, "Take your medications, dear, so that you will get well"–
or whether she was engaging in a form of passive suicide. Many dialysis
patients, not unlike most suicidal persons, experience a deep sense of
ambivalence about whether they want to live or die. Anger and Anger
(1974) write that:

> The patient on dialysis therapy exists as a part of two worlds–the
> world of the living and the world of the dying. Because of the quality
> of life he must live, being dependent upon a machine for his life, it
> becomes very difficult for him to decide which of the two worlds he
> wishes to become a part of. He thus is faced with a dilemma–fear of
> death and fear of life. (p. 30)

Strauss and Glaser (1975) suggest that "unresolved dependency conflicts
have been posited as contributory–if not causal–factors in the suicidal
despair of many renal failure patients, being directly related to the aggra-
vated problem of machine bondage" (p. 116). Strauss and Glaser indicate
that the dialysis patient's noncompliance with the medical regimen may be
a form of suicide. It is not surprising that "there is a significantly higher
incident of suicidal behavior among chronic renal patients than for the
general population at large, or even as compared with other chronic disease contexts" (Ibid., 116). I admired Maria's spunk for declaring war on a
system that creates dependency, which she feared would reduce her to the

compliant, listless, and submissive behavior of her fellow patients; yet I feared that her noncompliance, however noble, would inevitably result in an earlier death.

A crisis concerning Maria's emotional status and staff interaction appeared imminent. Maria's emotional health deteriorated rapidly as expressed by her poor appetite, irritability, and insomnia. It became necessary to work with the staff to lessen their resistance to alternative patient care approaches. She constantly criticized the medical staff for carelessly setting the pressure of the dialysis machine too high or forgetting to take her off dialysis at the designated time. Maria would then lapse into despondency and refuse to converse with the staff.

CASE CONFERENCE

A case conference seemed the best approach to seek solutions. I obtained authorization from the clinical director to conduct a combination in-service/patient staffing, and received approval from Maria to share her concerns with the staff. I selected an afternoon when fewer patients would be on the dialysis unit, thereby creating a relatively unstressful time for the staff. To avoid interruptions, we assembled in a conference room. Focusing on a team-approach strategy, I invited the six dialysis technicians, two RNs, four LPNs, and the two nephrologists involved in Maria's care. The staff's perception of Maria focused on her defiance of authority and noncompliance with the treatment regimen.

In part, my goal was to have the clinical staff consider such issues as independence and dependence. I told them how Maria had likened the dialysis machine to an umbilical cord and that she bitterly complained about feelings of helplessness and a loss of control. We then discussed ways of restoring some autonomy to Maria's life. One nurse suggested that Maria be allowed to take her own blood pressure, which Maria had once requested.

Several of the patients had expressed an interest in making plastercrafts during dialysis, and an arts and craft business owner had offered to instruct them on the process. With staff approval, I offered to submit a formal proposal to the hospital director to plan for this activity. The staff was enthusiastic. Working as a team and becoming united in a plan, the staff was pleased at their ability to contribute to Maria's well-being.

Maria had also indicated an interest in starting and editing a patient newsletter. The staff thought that this was a good idea and that the responsibility would establish a sense of accomplishment and autonomy in her life. Allowing Maria to check her own blood pressure, to become involved in the plastercraft program, and to edit a patient newsletter were ways in which she could regain a sense of control and independence, thereby helping to alleviate her depression and feelings of helplessness and worthlessness.

Frequently health care professionals feel guilty and defeated when they fail to accomplish their basic mission, that of healing. I attempted to elicit from the staff whether they shared these feelings. A spirited discussion followed on the importance of patients getting well. Most of the staff maintained that they work toward healing and curing at all costs, while some felt there was a time to die. The case conference provided a forum to discuss this issue and served as needed ventilation for the hospital staff. Holden (1980) contends that medical professionals are geared toward healing and curing their patients. She argues that uremic death for the dialysis patient should sometimes be seen as a viable alternative, but unfortunately "medical training does not prepare physicians to perceive the full range of alternatives and present them to clients" (p. 19).

Another issue that surfaced was related to Maria not comprehending many of the medical terms used casually by the staff. The nephrologist pointed out that the medical terminology associated with dialysis is complicated and that he was unsure if a substitute language existed, but that he would make an effort to explain to Maria in terms she could understand. The staff became aware of the anxiety and apprehension Maria felt when staff members evaded questions about her health. Maria shared with me that "she always fears the worst when people are not straight with her." Some of the staff seemed to understand the need to share medical information and agreed to be more open with her. Kubler-Ross (1974) writes that "a patient is much more frightened, much more anxious, and much more prone to difficulties if you are not honest with him" (p. 12).

One dialysis technician said that she seldom if ever talked about her feelings at home because "I'm a professional [sic], and I don't like to burden my family with all that goes on here." Kubler-Ross (1975) reports that:

> We also live in a society in which joining a profession is associated with something called 'professional behavior.' In either case, the showing of emotions, the sharing of feelings, and, particularly, the showing of such personal indicators as tears are taboos in our society, particularly for professionals and especially for males. The grieving patient, the patient who cries, not only makes us feel guilty, but he also makes us feel scared about our own ability to sustain a relationship without losing the mask identified with a professional stance. (p. 11)

As health care professionals whose objective is to help patients recover, it is uncomfortable when patients deteriorate physically, especially when dying has begun. Kalish (1985) asserts that:

> In some ways, they pay a penalty for this form of nurturing. On occasion, they develop relationships with the dying patients that are so close that they end up grieving when the patient dies. They think and talk about the dead person, feel helpless because of their inability to have changed his or her life course, may cry or feel depressed, and may even express displaced anger, anxiety, or difficulty in concentrating. Even such symptoms as fatigue, headaches, insomnia, and appetite loss are not uncommon (Lerea & LiMauro, 1982). In fact, they develop the familiar symptoms that all grieving people encounter. (p. 280)

I guided the discussion to the importance of seeing Maria within a cultural context, especially concerning food issues. Maria needed her mother to bring Mexican food because it symbolized the home she had left and her mother's expression of love for her. The nursing director said that hospital policy prohibited bringing in food but that the staff would relax the policy for occasional occurrences. Also, she would confer with the nutritionist about cooking more Mexican food. It was further recommended that the nutritionist and Maria's mother meet so low-sodium Mexican recipes, a requirement for dialysis patients, could be developed. Maria also requested she be given choices in her hospital meals. It was further agreed that Maria's eleven-year-old sister could visit in spite of hospital policy disallowing children visitations.

Both Maria and her mother felt that the hospital food was making her even sicker. Clark (1970) describes one newly arrived Mexican to the U.S. who attributed her poor health to the "artificial" food she ate (p. 201). Señora Garcia had once taken me aside to advise me that Maria is becoming weaker and "she's all skin and bone." In a hushed tone, she asked me, "Do you think that the doctors are poisoning Maria?" Maria later advised me that her mother had diagnosed her stomach problem as "Latido" in her stomach. Another time Señora Garcia diagnosed Maria's pain in her heart as "latida de corrazon" which Clark (1970) asserts is characterized by "high fever, pain and a cough" (p. 201). At the time Maria weighed 75 pounds. Señora Garcia would often sneak into Maria's room a large bowl of chicken broth covered with a large white cloth as a disguise. On more than one occasion I was also treated to chicken broth. "Oh, Miguel, you're looking so pale! Here, I have brought you some 'caldo'." Señora Garcia had requested permission to address me as Miguel which I considered indicative of her rapport with me. My ability to connect emotionally with the family was enhanced by my ability to communicate in Spanish.

I raised the issue of Maria's anger and depression and its relationship to the grieving process. I explained that Maria, like other patients who are having difficulty coping, directed her anger conveniently toward her caregivers. One of the nurses said that she understood the reasons for anger but "it's really difficult when it's directed right at you." Another nurse reminded the group that not taking patients' feelings personally is just part of being a professional. Rando (1986) urges caregivers to understand that such emotions as fear, anxiety, sadness, etc., are "hidden under the facade of anger" (p. 108). She writes that "verbalization of anger under most conditions must be understood and tolerated" (p. 110). DeSpelder and Strickland (1987) report that anger and outrage are typically expressed during the grieving process, and these feelings represent a reaction to the "injustice of the loss" (p. 210).

Maria became upset when scolded for not following medical directives—that is, she would have to take dialysis alone in the other room if she continued with her "emotional outbursts"; or when someone said "shame on you" when she didn't take her morning medications. One nurse shared a situation whereby Maria told her that she feels "like a 'bad girl' when you talk in that tone of voice. Until now, I didn't know what she meant."

One of the nurses said that she would see Maria occasionally reading one of Kubler-Ross' books. I pointed out that it was one way of answering questions about her dying—or finding out what questions she should ask.

Maria advised me that her mother was concerned because Señor Garcia was having difficulty sleeping and his appetite was poor. I related the importance of involving all family members in the treatment plan, especially the father who did not have a vehicle to ventilate his feelings and seemed struggling alone with his deep depression. I suggested that we all need to make ourselves available for discussions with family members when they visited, including discussions of a seemingly nonmedical nature.

One of the technicians thought it strange that, when Maria's family visited, there was a certain emotional commonality shared by all members; their expressions were stoic and absent affect. Rosen (1990) reports that in Phase 2 of anticipatory grieving, which he has termed "Living with Fatal Illness," the family has learned to cope by denying "any differences in temperament, emotions, and attitudes among family members" (p. 76). Rosen writes that "the family enters into an unspoken pact: We are all in this together, and we must all act and feel the same; we shall pretend to be alike" (p. 76). This behavior, termed "pseudomutuality," is potentially destructive because family members' emotions are repressed and turned inwardly, rather than expressed outwardly. The staff was made aware of the importance of not changing the subject when feelings were expressed; instead, the family members would be encouraged to express their feelings.

The case conference proved productive as demonstrated by the staff's willingness to implement the intervention strategies which are integrated into the treatment plan which follows.

TREATMENT PLAN

I. Regain a sense of autonomy, independence, control

Tasks for Maria:

A. To take her own blood pressure;

B. To edit a patient newsletter; and

C. To receive information about her medical condition and participate in decisions regarding her medical regimen.

Tasks for Staff:

A. Allow and encourage Maria and other patients to make plaster-crafts to market commercially;

B. Substitute confusing medical terminology (cliches and terms) for more understandable language when explaining medical information to Maria;

C. Explain and not "scold" or treat Maria punitively when she is in noncompliance with medical directives.

II. Help Maria through grieving process

Tasks for Staff:

A. Assist staff to develop effective (active) listening skills by not avoiding patient (or family) and changing the subject when she raises issues about death and dying;

B. Work toward coming to terms with staff members' mortality by freely discussing death and dying issues as they relate to themselves and to patients, i.e., staff would ventilate feelings in groups;

C. Accept expression of feelings and emotion, and to not take them personally;

D. Allow Maria access to death and dying literature.

III. Facilitate cultural sensitivity

Tasks for Staff

A. Treat the family as a unit by allowing and encouraging visitations of all family members (including grandparents, aunts, uncles, cousins, and her young sister) and friends;

B. Encourage Maria to share information on the cuarandero, Mexican fiestas, etc.;

C. Schedule a meeting between Maria's mother and the Anglo nutritionist to develop low-sodium recipes for Mexican foods;

D. Talk to the nutritionist about preparing more Mexican foods and providing a menu to Maria for selection;

E. Involve family members in the overall treatment plan by:

   1. Arranging for scheduled times when Maria's mother can bring in Mexican food;

   2. Encouraging open communication between Maria and her father.

Treatment Plan Assessment (Six-Months Following Implementation)

With the authorization of the clinical director and encouragement from the medical staff, Maria, together with 41 other patients, had received training in constructing plastercrafts. Much of Maria's time became dedicated to the production and marketing of plastercrafts. The Renal Care Unit was transformed into a radiant, electrifying atmosphere. Unlike the gloom that once pervaded, there was a sense of community with Maria as the editor of the *Renal Review* energetically gathering patient and staff "tidbits."

"I'm now the only one who takes my blood pressure!" Maria proudly exclaimed. Not only did Maria feel more in control, but there was instilled a sense of importance as the medical staff began sharing information with her. Maria confided in me that she would always expect the worst "when they'd hide medical information from me, but now they let me know exactly how I'm doing and I'm starting to understand more about what they're saying."

A dialysis technician shared with me that she read a book on death and dying written by Kubler-Ross that Maria had lent her: "After I read it, Maria quizzed me on specific points. When it was obvious that I'd missed a key point, she was sure to correct me. I guess that the next time I read anything she recommends, I'll read it for detail."

The medical staff and I began working on developing deeper relationships with Maria's family members, especially her father. Whenever the family members visited Maria, I would usually see them conversing with dialysis staff members. Staff noticed that family visits increased and that even her father was visiting Maria more regularly. "I think that maybè he accepts that I'm not going to get well," a relieved Maria remarked as if to convey that finally she could die in peace. Family members would return faithfully every day to maintain an all-day vigil. There appeared to be a sense of resignation that Maria was soon to die. Señora Garcia reminded Maria to continue drinking her "caldo" because it was making her stronger, and that soon she would be able to visit the family for a week-end visit, but she seemed to lack conviction in what she was saying. Rosen (1990) has identified Phase 3 in anticipatory grieving as that of Final Acceptance. "It is not unusual at this stage for one person to be making funeral plans while another continues to insist that the patient is looking better every day" (p. 77). It was apparent that Maria's condition had deteriorated rapidly. She weighed 65 pounds and it was an enormous effort just for her to talk. No longer was she seen scurrying about the unit, she was now confined to a bed. Maria's outbursts of anger had subsided and she seemed to be coming to terms with her dying, due in part to a now openly communicative medical staff who talked freely with her about her concerns.

Soon thereafter Maria died. Unlike other dialysis patients who receive scant recognition upon their death, Maria was described variously by the staff as "having spunk and courage." Octavio Paz (Irish et al., 1993), the celebrated Mexican writer, seemed to describe Maria when he talked about

> ... the need to confront death, the need to not be afraid, the need to always be ready to die, and the need to never give in, but rather to welcome death whenever it comes, whatever its form, and whatever the reason. (p. 74)

Just before she died, Maria asserted proudly, "As far as I'm concerned, death is something I look forward to."

REFERENCES

Anger, D., & Anger, D. (1974). Life in the balance. *Dialysis and Transplantation, June-July,* 30-32.

Beechem, M. (videotaped communication, April 3, 1975).

Cassell, E. J. (1974). Dying in a technological society. *Hastings Center Studies, 2* (2), 31-35.

Clark, M. (1970). *Health in the Mexican-American culture.* Los Angeles: University of California Press.

Cowgill, D. O. (1986). *Aging around the world*. Belmont, CA: Wadsworth Publishing Company.

De La Rosa, M. (1989). Health care needs of Hispanic Americans and the responsiveness of the health care system. *Health and Social Work, May 1989*, 104-113.

DeSpelder, L. A., & Strickland, A. L. (1987). *The last dance: Encountering death and dying*. Mountainview, CA: Mayfield Publishing Company.

Falicov, C. J. (1982). Mexican families. In M. McGoldrick, J. K. Pearce, & J. Giordano (Eds.), *Ethnicity and family therapy*. New York: Guilford Press.

Holden, M. O. (1980). Dialysis or death: The ethical alternative. *Health and Social Work. 5* (2), 19.

Hyland, J. M. (1978). The role of denial in the patient with cancer. Presentations at the Forum for Death Education and Counseling, Washington, D.C.

Kalish, R. (1985). *Death, grief and caring relationships*. Monterey, CA: Brooks/Cole Publishing Company.

Kubler-Ross, E. (1974). *Questions and answers on death and dying*. New York: Collier Books.

Kubler-Ross, E. (1975). *Death: The final state of growth*. Englewood Cliffs, NJ: Prentice-Hall, Inc.

Lerea, L. E. & LiMauro, B. F. (1982). Grief among healthcare workers: A comparative study. *Journal of Gerontology. 37*, 604-608.

Lewis, O. (1959). *Five families*. New York: Basic Books.

McGoldrick, M., Pearce, J. and Giordano, J. (1982). *Ethnicity and Family Therapy*. NY: Guilford Press.

Parkes, C. M. (1981). Sudden death and its impact on the family. In J. Schneider, *Stress, loss, & grief*. Baltimore: University Park Press.

Paz, O. (1993). In Irish, D. P., Lundquist, K. F., & Nelson, V. J. (Eds.). *Ethnic variations in dying, death, and grief: Diversity in universality*. Washington, D.C.: Taylor & Francis.

Ramirez, R. (personal communication, August 30, 1993).

Rando, T. A. (1986). *Loss and anticipatory grief*. Lexington, Mass: Lexington Books.

Rosen, E. (1990). *Families facing death: Family dynamics of terminal illness*. Lexington, MA: Lexington Books.

Schneider, J. (1984). *Stress, loss and grief: Understanding their origins and growth potential*. Baltimore: University Park Press.

Seligman, M. E. P. (1975). *Helplessness: On depression, development and death*. San Francisco: W. H. Freeman.

Sotomayor, M. (1989). The Hispanic elderly and the intergenerational family. *The Journal of Children in Contemporary Society. 20, 55-65*.

Strauss, A. L., & Glaser, B. G. (1975). *Chronic illness and the quality of life*. St. Louis: The C. V. Mosley Co.

Trevino, E. (1984). *Health Indicators for Hispanic, Black, and White Americans*. DHHS Publication No. 84-1576, Washington, D.C.: U.S. Government Printing Office.

Hispanic American Elders: Caregiving Norms Surrounding Dying and the Use of Hospice Services

Melissa A. Talamantes
W. Ross Lawler
David V. Espino

SUMMARY. The purpose of this review is to (1) provide an over-view of health and demographic characteristics common to the Hispanic elder population, (2) address family caregiving issues surrounding the terminal illness of a loved one, (3) understand re-source utilization by Hispanic elderly and their family caregivers, and (4) make recommendations for the provision of information and education about hospice services. Case examples will illustrate patterns and themes unique to Hispanic caregiving. *[Single or multiple copies of this article are available from The Haworth Document Delivery Service: 1-800-342-9678, 9:00 a.m. - 5:00 p.m. (EST).]*

BACKGROUND

The Hispanic elderly represent a large and ethnically-diverse part of the Hispanic population. Subgroups which are classified under "Hispanic"

Melissa A. Talamantes, MS, W. Ross Lawler, MD, and David V. Espino, MD, are from the Department of Family Practice, University of Texas Health Science Center, San Antonio, TX.

Address all correspondence to: Melissa A. Talamantes, MS, Department of Family Practice, 7703 Floyd Curl Dr., San Antonio, TX 78284-7795.

[Haworth co-indexing entry note]: "Hispanic American Elders: Caregiving Norms Surrounding Dying and the Use of Hospice Services." Talamantes, Melissa A., W. Ross Lawler, and David V. Espino. Co-published simultaneously in *The Hospice Journal* (The Haworth Press, Inc.) Vol. 10, No. 2, 1995, pp. 35-49; and: *Hospice Care and Cultural Diversity* (ed: Donna Lind Infeld, Audrey K. Gordon, and Bernice Catherine Harper) The Haworth Press, Inc., 1995, pp. 35-49. Single or multiple copies of this article are available from The Haworth Document Delivery Service: [1-800-342-9678, 9:00 a.m. - 5:00 p.m. (EST)].

35

are the Mexican Americans, Puerto Ricans, Cubans, and Central and South Americans. Each of these ethnic groups has a distinctive socio-historical background, unique cultural norms and patterns of interaction, and are concentrated in various regions of the United States.

According to the Bureau of the Census (1991), Hispanic elders (age 65 and older) represent 5.1 percent of the total Hispanic population. The origins of this Hispanic American elder cohort consist of 54 percent Mexican, 10 percent Puerto Rican, 14 percent Cuban, 8 percent Central or South American and 13 percent classified as other Hispanic elderly. The Hispanic elderly average five years of formal education and have the second highest illiteracy rate among all racial/ethnic groups. Approximately 90 percent of Hispanic elderly speak Spanish in their homes. Although 22 percent report that they do not speak any English, 50 percent speak English well (U.S. Bureau of the Census, 1977).

The level of financial security of the Hispanic elderly is poor. In 1986, the median annual income for elderly Hispanic men was $7,369, and for elderly Hispanic women was $4,583 (Bureau of Labor Statistics, 1987). In 1991, the Bureau of the Census reported that 17 percent of Hispanic elderly were below the poverty level. One-third of Hispanic elders are covered by Medicare and Medicaid, 21 percent have Medicare and private insurance, 28 percent have only Medicare, 10 percent have other insurance, and 8 percent do not have any health insurance (Schick, 1991).

The magnitude of health problems affecting Hispanic elderly is great, but health-related data is scant. The Hispanic Health and Nutrition Examination Survey (HHANES) was conducted from 1982-84. Secondary analysis of this data revealed that older Hispanics who were least acculturated were at greater risk for the development of hypertension (Espino et al., 1990). The leading causes of death for Hispanic elders include ischemic heart disease, malignant neoplasms, cerebrovascular disease, chronic pulmonary obstructive disease, pneumonia and influenza, and diabetes mellitus. Hispanic elderly are almost twice as likely as the general elder population to have more than one limitation in activities of daily living (ADLs) (bathing, toileting, dressing, eating, transferring) and instrumental activities of daily living (IADLs) (housework, shopping, meal preparation, managing money) (Schick et al., 1991). Sotomayor and colleagues (1988) reported that they required assistance with IADLs more often than needing help with ADLs. Mental health problems affecting the Hispanic elderly must also be addressed. In a community-based study of Mexican American elderly, researchers found that 26 percent suffered from depression and dysphoria. This rate increased when associated with a medical disability. None of these elderly were receiving appropriate medical treatment or other services for their illness (Kemp et al. 1987). Similarly, Mintzer et al. (1992) found that Cuban American elders had a higher incidence of symptoms of depression compared with non-Hispanic white elderly.

Hispanic elderly tend to live in the community and are less likely to utilize long-term care institutions (Espino, 1988). For the Mexican American elderly cohort, studies show substantial intergenerational support between elders and their children (Markides, 1986). The Hispanic community continues to provide informal familial support to their elderly family members (Sotomayor, 1992; Greene & Monahan, 1984; Cox & Gelfand, 1987; Keefe et. al, 1979). However, controversy exists over whether familial support systems remain strong or whether they are eroding as a result of changing economics, mobility, and lifestyles (Jimenez-Velasquez, 1992; Rothman, 1992; Newton & Ruiz, 1980). Table 1 presents the living arrangements of elderly Hispanic males and females compared with non-Hispanic whites.

HISPANIC FAMILY CAREGIVING

Although research on Hispanic caregivers is sparse, a few studies have addressed the psychological status of Hispanic caregivers. Cox and Monk (1990) found that Hispanic caregivers had higher levels of depression than African American caregivers. In fact, the mean score on the Center for Epidemiological Scale for Depression (CES-D) was 20 for Hispanic caregivers, exceeding the usual cutoff score of 16 for depression.

TABLE 1

Living Arrangements of
Hispanic and Non-Hispanic White Elderly

	HISPANIC			NON-HISPANIC WHITE
	Total	Men	Women	Total
Alone	19%	11%	25%	31%
With Spouse	51%	73%	36%	56%
With Other Relatives	27%	14%	36%	11%
With Non-Relatives Only	3%	2%	3%	2%

Source: U.S. Bureau of the Census, 1992

Although there are many cross-cultural variations, the literature suggests that families provide high levels of support to Hispanic elders in time of need (Wallace & Lew-Ting, 1992; Lubben & Becerra, 1987; Delgado, 1982). The idea of "filial piety" (moral obligation of children to care for and respect elders) may be a common reason for continued familial assistance to Hispanic elderly (Cox & Gelfand, 1987). Markides' (1986) three-generational study of Mexican Americans found that elders had high unfulfilled expectations of their children.

Level of acculturation helps us to understand differences in communication patterns, interactional behaviors, role performances, cultural norms, values, and behaviors among various individuals and groups. Researchers have described different levels of acculturation in relation to the "acculturation continuum" (Gordon, 1964; Valle, 1989). At one end of this continuum are traditional beliefs and affiliations with the culture of origin. In the middle is bicultural orientation where one is able to move from their traditional culture to the mainstream host society with little difficulty. At the other end, assimilated persons have left their own cultural roots and now identify with the host society. The Hispanic elderly may remain closer to the traditional side of the continuum. For example, they may speak Spanish only and prefer traditional ethnic foods. Family caregivers' beliefs about the delivery of care to their elderly family members depend on individual and group values inherent in each ethnic group. Caregivers may be at various positions along this acculturation continuum which may be a source of tension if they are not at the same level as their elderly family members.

As suggested by Valle (1989), Hispanic caregivers often fall into the category of bicultural. However, they may "revert to traditional modes in deference to their elder family member." Unfortunately, most caregiver studies have failed to include ethnic values and beliefs as variables for examining illnesses, stress, and burden (Hernandez, 1991).

HISPANIC ELDERS' USE OF HEALTH AND SOCIAL SERVICES

Hispanic elders used senior centers and benefitted by meals provided by senior centers more than any other service in 1988 (Schick & Schick, 1991). Home health aides were used by only 5 percent of elders while 7 percent used home-delivered meals and homemaker services, 9 percent had visiting nurses, and 12 percent used transportation services (Ibid.).

Wallace's earlier study (1982) revealed that acculturation did not significantly correlate with the use of home health care services by Hispanic elders. He suggests that structural forces such as health insurance and living arrangements influenced their elders' use of home health care services. The absence of private insurance for Mexican Americans significantly limited access to medical care (Wells et al., 1988). Based on another study, of 704 Hispanics over age 60, 79 percent sought care from a primary care physician during the previous year, regardless of their ability to speak English (Lopez-Aqueres et al., 1984). However, this finding was based on a sample in a large city with a substantial Hispanic community. Underutilization of services by Hispanic elders could be attributed to alienation. Discrimination and prejudice inherent in their socio-historical backgrounds may have caused suspicion and mistrust of the formal service sector (Purdy & Arguello, 1992). Finally, language barriers, lack of awareness of existing services, lack of availability of culturally-sensitive services, and lack of perceived need for services are factors which may also contribute to the underutilization of health and social services by Hispanic elderly (Starrett et al., 1983).

ETHNOCULTURAL THEMES TO CAREGIVING, DYING, AND DEATH

Race, ethnicity, culture, religion, spirituality, family dynamics, socio-economic status, and education level are some of the factors that may affect one's perceptions and beliefs about illness, suffering, pain, coping, dying, and death. The norms and rituals surrounding the process of dying and death are culturally bound in attitudes and beliefs passed on from generation to generation.

There is little data describing the attitude of family caregivers from various ethnic/cultural groups toward the provision of care for terminally ill family members. Most studies discuss ethnic/racial differences between African American and Euroanglo respondents concerning their attitudes about dying at home versus in a hospital, and accepting hospice care. One study found that 62 percent of African Americans would prefer to die in their home rather than in the hospital, whereas 81 percent of Euroanglos prefer to die at home (Neubauer & Hamilton, 1990).

In a study of hospice users from St. Luke's/Roosevelt Palliative Care Service, an inner city program in New York City, 14 percent of recipients of care were Hispanic compared to 58 percent Black and 28 percent White. Ethnic/racial differences in utilization of services at the St. Luke's program and in the New York State Hospice Association were great. Of those utilizing hospice services, 2 percent were Hispanic, 6 percent were Black, and 92 percent were non-Hispanic White (Pawling-Kaplan & O'Connor, 1989).

One reason for low service utilization by Hispanics may be related to provider referral. Physicians may play a large role in brokering services to elderly and their families (Wallace & Lew-Ting, 1992). In this particular situation, physicians may not refer Hispanic patients to a hospice because they "observe families providing in-home support and assume that such assistance is provided for cultural reasons" (Ibid.).

The literature suggests that socioeconomic factors such as income and education levels, lack of health insurance, an absence of awareness about available services, and previous negative experiences in accessing medical and social services may be contributing to the lower use of formal services by Hispanic elderly (Trevino, 1988, De la Rosa, 1989, Wells et al., 1988). Sotomayor and Randolph (1988) posit that other variables which contribute to the Hispanic elderly's reduced ability to access and utilize health care services include: language, gender, time of immigration (if immigrated), level of acculturation, proximity to mother country, and generational position on the continuum of migration. Although research suggests no major differences in the use of inpatient medical services among Mexican Americans and non-Hispanic whites (Wells et al., 1988), higher socioeconomic levels increase the use of outpatient services more by non-Hispanic whites than among Mexican Americans. Lopez-Aqueres and colleagues (1984) found in their study of elderly Mexican Americans that language was associated with the type of physician seen. Those elders who were Spanish speaking only tended to see primary care physicians and those who spoke English were more likely seen by specialists. The elderly cohort of Hispanics who may either be fluent in Spanish only or bilingual, however prefer to communicate in Spanish, still face sociocultural barriers which prevent them from seeking health care services.

Illness perceptions of Hispanic elderly, stemming from their cultural belief systems, are important determinants of the help-seeking process for hospice services. Cox (1986) found that 38 percent of elderly Hispanics attributed their health problems to old age. Serious health complications can occur if elderly wait too long before seeking health care. These elderly Hispanics also reported having a supportive relationship with their physician. Rothman (1992) discussed the fear of terminal illness among elderly Cuban-Americans which prevents them from seeking health care services. He suggested that elderly Cuban-Americans have a fatalistic belief that there is no solution or remedy to prevent the onset of a terminal illness. This belief may explain their use of denial as a coping strategy. This supports the study by Wallace (1992) indicating that physicians may be key as service brokers. Since physicians are the primary referral source to hospice services, more research is needed to determine the relationship of race/ethnicity and family caregiving patterns as they affect physician referrals.

Perceptions of death within Hispanic cultures can be viewed from socio-historical perspectives. Rael and Korte (1988), in their qualitative study on Hispanics in New Mexico, discuss the cyclical relationship between life and death. They describe the writings of Paz in which he poignantly talks about "life flowing into death, its opposite and complement; and death in turn, was not an end in itself."

For those Mexican Americans who have maintained cultural ties to Mexico, celebrations and festivals are common. In order to understand customs and cultural beliefs, it is essential to know the historical background of each ethnic group. A traditional celebration in Mexico, "*Dia de los Muertos,*" or "Day of the Dead," is similar to the pre-Columbian "Day of the Dead" and the European-Catholic "All Souls Day." In North America, many regions with large Mexican American populations celebrate this occasion with "Dia de los Muertos" parades and festivals. In addition, families visit the graves of those who have died before them. Museums often organize art displays with altars honoring the dead.

Rael and Korte's (1988) cultural analysis of the rural communities in northern New Mexico found that "death" is a natural part of life in the community throughout the year. For example, offering masses in honor of the anniversary of a family member's death is a common occurrence. Publishing a paragraph in a local newspaper with semipoetic material remembering a loved one's death is also common. This is not unique to Hispanics in New Mexico (Ibid.). In the Catholic church, parishioners offer masses daily or light candles in honor of someone who has died. In addition, many Catholics believe that deceased family members are "watching over them" in times of difficulty. They pray to them for continued support and strength.

Death is a recurring theme in Mexican fictional literature (Younoszai, 1993) and is often represented in the work of the famous Mexican artist, Frida Kahlo, who is only recently receiving recognition for her paintings about her own suffering and dying. Many other writers and artists use the theme of dying and death as an integral part of their work.

Hispanic folk healing systems are as diverse as each ethnic group. Espiritismo is practiced in Puerto Rico, Mexico, and other countries and consists of communication by espiritistas (spiritual healers) with "spirits" for purposes of purifying an ill person's soul. The belief in Santeros (Cuban faith healers) and the practice of Santeria (the healing of evil spirits) for spiritual guidance and healing has its origins in the Cuban/Dominican communities and is based on African traditions. The equivalent of this healer in Mexico is the curandero (general practitioner of Mexican folk healing). Other folk healers may include yerbistas (herbalists), soba-dores (massage therapists), and others based on various Latin American countries and ethnic groups (Cuellar, 1990). Often Hispanic elderly are stereotyped as preferring these folk healers to Western medical providers. A recognition that these forms of healers exist is important, but to what extent each Hispanic elder group and their families utilize them is not known. The following cases illustrate the relationship between cultural themes or patterns underlying the beliefs and values among Hispanic caregivers and the care they provide to loved ones with terminal illnesses.

CASE #1

Mrs. L. was a 68 year old Mexican American woman who immigrated to the U.S. in the early 1930s from Mexico. Mrs. L. was bilingual; how-ever, she preferred to communicate in Spanish. She had Parkinson's dis-ease and, although she had many physical limitations, she was the co-pri-mary caregiver with her husband for her 90 year-old mother, Mrs. S., an end stage diabetic. This couple had three adult children, two who lived in close proximity and provided instrumental and emotional support for their parents. Mrs. L. said she could ask for help from her children for trans-portation or other needs, however she did not want to "take advantage of them because they had their families and their own problems." She rarely discussed her fears and worries about her mother's deterioration or about her own illness. Mrs. S had both lower extremities amputated and required total care. A home health care agency provided a home health aide for Mrs. S.'s personal care.

Mrs. L. became known to the social service agency when she heard a radio program in Spanish on memory problems. She reported that her mother had been experiencing memory problems for the past three years and her behavior had become significantly worse. Mrs. S.'s physician told Mr. and Mrs. L. that it was related to old age. Mrs. L. said, "Dios es grande, pienso que los problemas de la memoria de mi Mamá son debidos a alguna enfermedad" (God is great, and I believe that her memory prob-lems are related to some disease). As she was arranging for a memory evaluation for her mother, Mrs. S. had a massive stroke and died. On the day of her funeral, Mr. L. also had a massive stroke and was left in a coma in intensive care.

Mrs. L. felt physically very bad because of the Parkinson's. She cried constantly and reported that she did not feel up to going out of her house. Throughout the duration of his hospitalization, she reported never losing hope for his recovery. She didn't discuss his possible death with his doctor or their children. "I talked to him every time I visited and would let him know how things were going, I told him that he is going to get better." "Yo ruego a Dios que lo alivie de su sufrimiento y que se alivia" (I pray to God to heal his suffering and to heal him).

Mrs. L. mentioned to the nurse her concern about his toe having some discoloration. The nurse checked his toe but indicated that it was not serious. A few days later, Mr. L. had a fever and his leg was cyanotic. The doctors advised Mrs. L. that they would have to amputate his leg. Two days later, after the surgery, Mr. L. died. Mrs. L. had never given up hope for his recovery.

CASE #2

Mrs. D. was a 78 year old Cuban American who was caring for her 80 year old husband in the end stages of probable Alzheimer's Disease. They had two adult children who live in the same city, however not in close proximity. Mrs. D. spoke limited English and was referred to the social service agency by an Adult Day Health Center located two blocks away. Members of the center had tried many times to help Mrs. D., however she repeatedly refused any outside help. She said, "No tengo confianza en personas que no conozco" (I don't trust people that I don't know).

Mr. D. required total care and Mrs. D. had one friend who came to her house to bathe and transfer him to the wheelchair each morning. The friend returned in the evening to transfer Mr. D. back to bed. Mrs. D. said that she prayed daily for strength to help her keep going as she worried about her own health. She was very upset as she reminisced about over 50 years with her husband. She described their relationship as being very close and they functioned as a team. "Compartimos el café de la misma taza" (We share coffee from the same cup).

Talking about his death was difficult and she said that she would prefer to suffer the burden of caring for him the way he was than not having him around at all. She said that living in the U.S. was so different from living in Cuba or any Latin American country. "Here the children live far away and work all day; everyone is busy. In Cuba, there would always be someone around to help or just to check in–a niece, cousin, aunt." Although she could rely on her son, she did not want to impose on him because he had an important job. Mrs. D. was very tearful and said that she never expected her husband to get this disease. "Yo rezo mis oraciones a diario, mi fé es en Dios, porque Dios es poderoso" (I say my daily prayers, I have faith in God because he is powerful).

CASE #3

Mrs. J. is a 54 year old Puerto Rican who cared for her 65 year old husband with end stage Amyotrophic Lateral Sclerosis (Lou Gehrig's Disease). Mr. J. had this disease for about 15 years, however only in the past four years had his health begun to deteriorate. Throughout the course of his illness, Mr. J. had been seen by several neurologists in Puerto Rico and North America. Mrs. J's relatives brought over an "espiritista" (spiritual healer) to rid Mr. J. of "evil spirits." Mrs. J. said that later these espiritistas realized that her husband did not have evil spirits but rather a serious disease.

Mrs. J. had four children, two who lived in Puerto Rico. These adult children provided minimal support; Mrs. J. reported "Tienen sus familias y sus problemas, no pueden ayudar" (They have their families and their problems, they can't help). Although Mr. J. expressed a wish not to be on a respirator and to die at home with his family, they could not comply with his wish when he could no longer breathe and they saw him suffering too much. Eventually, Mr. J.'s lung collapsed. He was taken to the emergency room and put on a respirator. Eventually, he was discharged with a portable respirator. A neighbor (who had four children of her own) spent the nights with Mrs. J. and provided significant help with the total care he required. "Pedia a Dios que me seguiera ayudando" (I prayed to God to continue to help me). "Dios pide mucho y Dios ayuda mucho." Mrs. J. was tearful as she talked about her husband. She reported feeling nervous and having problems sleeping and eating. "Dios pide mucho y Dios ayuda mucho." (God asks for much and God gives much.) Mr. J.'s health worsened and he developed a fever. He was taken to the emergency room and admitted with pneumonia. Mrs. J.'s brother who was a physician advised her to prepare herself for his death. Mrs. J. could not believe that he was in the end stages of death. "Yo creia que el no iba morir porque tenia el ultimo modelo de maquina para respirar, Yo todavia tenia esperanza que iba a mejorar pero ya estaba muy malo" (I did not believe that he was going to die as he had the newest respirator. I still had hope that he would get better but he was very sick).

DISCUSSION

Some of the themes that emerge in reviewing these cases relate to religion, spirituality, and the similarities in the faith and hope these three caregivers displayed. Although the women came from different countries and had different cultural perspectives, there were similarities in their views toward service use, caregiving, filial expectations, dying, and death.

First, all mentioned having children available to help. However, only Mrs. L.'s children were actually providing instrumental support. The other caregivers felt that they could not rely on their children for support and emphasized not wanting to "burden or impose" on them. They never directly expressed beliefs about their children's obligation to help them. However, one caregiver alluded to the differences between Cuban and American families regarding providing support. All of these women were primary caregivers and two of them received extensive support from informal non-family supportive networks. Only one, whose mother was receiving home-health care and whose husband was in an acute care setting, received any formal help. This supports the finding that the availability of informal care reduces the probability of receiving formal care and also affects the caregiver's decision about relying on formal care (Kemper, 1992). All the caregivers exhibited depressive symptomology which has been reported in previous caregiving literature on Hispanic caregivers (Cox & Monk, 1990).

It appeared that coping strategies in dealing with caregiving responsibilities and terminal illness included faith and hope. Their "dichos" (sayings) related to prayer and relying on God as the "all powerful and all knowing" were present constantly. In interviews conducted with northern New Mexicans, many used similar "dichos" about God, faith, and spirituality (Rael & Korte, 1988). It is not understood how much of this faith and hope are aspects of their religious upbringing, their family traditions and beliefs, or part of their continued spiritual growth. Whatever the roots and origins of this faith, it is evident that on some level it has helped them to cope with the stresses of caregiving, the dying, and the death of their loved ones.

RECOMMENDATIONS

If physicians do not refer Hispanic elderly to hospices or other health and social services, then it is essential that hospices initiate outreach measures to educate them and their family caregivers about available services. Recommendations for the provision of hospice information and education include to target educational programs to Hispanic family caregivers and agencies currently serving the Hispanic community. Hospice programs should actively seek out agencies currently providing services to the Hispanic community to conduct presentations about hospice care to staff and recipients of services. The focus of these presentations can serve three purposes: (1) educate the key community agency staff; (2) educate recipients of community services; and (3) recruit hospice volunteers. Recruiting individuals from the Hispanic community will increase the numbers of volunteers with bilingual or Spanish language capabilities and who are familiar with Hispanic cultural issues.

Active outreach interventions by hospice agencies may increase the community awareness of hospice providers and increase the numbers of linkages in the Hispanic community to people who could then refer individuals to hospice. Increasing the numbers of bilingual or Spanish language volunteers will greatly facilitate the placement of volunteers who can then communicate with patients and families and help decrease some of the cultural barriers to receiving care.

The second recommendation is to develop educational materials using various media (written, audiovisual). Educational materials should not be limited to translation of brochures into Spanish. Various levels of materials are needed (i.e., audiovisual, fotonovelas [picture books]) that can address all literacy levels.

Recommendation three is to actively recruit volunteers representing various Hispanic ethnic communities. By increasing the numbers of bilingual and bicultural volunteers, hospice agencies begin the necessary steps toward organizational diversity. Each organization should examine its board of directors and advisory councils to ensure its members represent the population needing services (in this case the Hispanic community). Active recruiting and hiring of bilingual and bicultural hospice providers will help the organization become more diverse. In addition, hospice organizations should provide cultural competency training to hospice staff.

Finally, reporting ethnicity as part of the National Home and Hospice Care Survey will ensure adequate data is available for future research and outreach endeavors. The development of a grass-roots approach to service delivery may increase the referrals from the Hispanic community for needed services. These recommendations will ensure the provision of hospice services reflect the cultural diversity of values inherent in the various Hispanic ethnic groups.

REFERENCES

Cox, C. (1986). Physician utilization by three groups of ethnic elderly. *Medical Care,* 24 (8): 667-676.

Cox, C. & Gelfand, D.E. (1987). Familial assistance, exchange and satisfaction among hispanic, portuguese, and vietnamese ethnic elderly. *Journal of Cross-Cultural Gerontology,* 2:241-255.

Cox, C. & Monk, A. (1990). Minority caregivers of dementia victims: a comparison of black and hispanic families. *Journal of Applied Gerontology, 9* (3):340-54.

Cuellar, J. (1990). Ethnogeriatric review: state of the literature summary. *Hispanic American Elders*. SGEC Working paper Series No. 5. Stanford, California: Stanford Geriatric Education Center.

De La Rosa, M. (1989). Health care needs of hispanic americans and the responsiveness of the health care system. *National Association of Social Workers, Inc.*, May 104-113.

Delgado, M. (1982). Ethnic and cultural variations in the care of the aged hispanic elderly and natural support systems: a special focus on Puerto Ricans. *Journal of Geriatric Psychiatry, 15*: 239-51.

Espino, D.V. (1990). Mexican american elderly: problems in evaluation, diagnosis, and treatment. In Harper MS (Ed). *Minority Aging: Essential Curricula Content for Selected Health and Allied Health Professionals*. Washington DC, PHS.

Espino, D.V., Neufeld, R.R., Mulvahill, M.K. (1988). Hispanic and non-Hispanic elderly on admission to the nursing home: a pilot study. *The Gerontologist, 28*:821-824.

Garcia, J.M. & Montgomery, P.A. (1991). The Hispanic population in the United States. Washington, D.C.: U.S. Department of Commerce, Bureau of the Census.

Gordon, M.M. (1964). *Assimilation in American life*. New York: Oxford Press.

Greene, V.L., & Monahan, D.J. (1984). Comparative utilization of community based long term care services by Hispanic and Anglo elderly in a case management system. *Journal of Gerontology, 39*(6):730-735.

Hernandez, G.G. (1991). Not so benign neglect: researchers ignore ethnicity in defining family caregiver burden and recommending services. Letters to the Editors. *The Gerontologist, 31*(2):271-272.

Jimenez-Velasquez, I.Z. (1992). Health and social issues concerning Puerto Rican elderly: a comparison between the New York and Puerto Rico experiences. In *Hispanic Aging: Research Reports Part I and II. National Institutes of Health, National Institute on Aging*.

Keefe, S.E., Padilla, A.M., & Carlos, M.C. (1979). The American extended family as an emotional support system. *Human Organization, 38*, 144-152.

Kemp, B.J., Staples, F. & Lopez-Agueres, W. (1987). Epidemiology of depression and dysphoria in an elderly Hispanic population. *Journal of the American Geriatric Society, 35*:920-926.

Kemper, P. (1992). The use of formal and informal home care by the disabled elderly. *Health Services Research, October, 27*(4),421-451.

Lopez-Agueres, W., Kemp, B., Staples, F. & Brummel-Smith, K. (1984). Use of health care services by older Hispanics. *Journal of the American Geriatrics Society, 32*(6):435-440.

Lubben, J.E., & Beccerra, R. (1987). Social support among black, Mexican and Chinese elderly. In D. Gelfund and C. Barresi, eds., *Ethnic Dimensions of Aging*. New York: Springer.

Markides, K.S., Boldt, J.S. & Ray, L.A. (1986). Sources of helping and intergenerational solidarity: a three-generations study of Mexican Americans. *Journal of Gerontology, 41*:506-511.

Mintzer, J.E., Rubert, M. P., Loewenstein, D., Gamez, E., Millor, A., Quinteros, R., Flores, L. Miller, M. Rainerman, A. & Eisdorfer, C. (1992). Daughters caregiving for Hispanic and non-Hispanic alzheimer patients: does ethnicity make a difference? *Community Mental Health Journal, 28*(4):293-303.

Newton, F. C-R. & Ruiz, R.A. (1980). Chicano culture and mental health. In *Chicano Aging and Mental Health*, M. Mirande & R. Ruiz (eds.) Rockville, MD: National Institute of Mental Health.

Neubauer, B. J. & Hamilton, C. L. (1990). Racial differences in attitudes toward hospice care. *Hospice Journal 6*(1):37-48.

Pawling-Kaplan, M. & O'Connor, P. (1989). Hospice care for minorities: an analysis of a hospital-based inner city palliative care service. *American Journal of Hospice Care 6*(4):13-21.

Purdy, J. K. & Arguello, D. (1992). Hispanic familism in caretaking of older adults: is it functional? *Journal of Gerontological Social Work, 19*(2):29-43.

Rael, R. & Korte, A.O. (1988). "El ciclo de la vida y muerte: an analysis of health and dying selected Hispanic enclave. In *Hispanic Elderly in Transition, Theory, Research Policy and Practice*. Ed. S. Applewhite. Greenwood Press, 189-202.

Rothman, S.M. (1992). Developing strategies for information dissemination to older Cuban Americans in Florida. In *Hispanic Aging: Research Reports Part I and II. National Institutes of Health, National Institute on Aging*.

Saluter, A.F. (1992). Marital status and living arrangements. Washington, D.C.: Department of Commerce, Bureau of the Census.

Schick, F.L. & Schick, R. (1991). *Statistical handbook on U.S. Hispanics*. Phoenix, Arizona: Oryx Press.

Sotomayor, M. (1992). Social support networks. In *Hispanic Aging: Research Reports Part I and II. National Institute of Health, National Institute on Aging*.

Sotomayor, M. & Randolph, S. (1988). Review of caregiving issues among Hispanic elderly: a cultural signature. In *Hispanic Elderly*. Edinburg: Pan American University Press.

Starett, R.A., Mindel, C.H., & Wright, R. (1983). Influence of support systems on the use of social services by the Hispanic elderly. *Social Work Research and Abstracts, 19*:35-40.

Treviño, M.C. (1988). A comparitive analysis of need, access, and utilization of health and human services. In *Hispanic Elderly in Transition: Theory, Research, Policy and Practice*. Greenwood Press Inc., 61-72.

U.S. Government Printing Office (1977). Persons of Spanish origin in the U.S. *U.S. Bureau of the Census Current Population Reports*. Series P-26, No. 361, Washington, D.C.

U.S. Government Printing Office (1987a and 1991b). The Hispanic population in the United States: March 1986 and 1987 (Advance Reports). *U.S. Bureau of the Census: Current Population Reports.* Series P-20, No. 416, Washington, D.C. 1-15.

U.S. Department of Labor (1987). Current population survey. *U.S. Bureau of Labor Statistics,* Washington, D.C.

U.S. Department of Health and Human Services (1992). The use of formal and informal home care by the disabled. *Agency for Health Care Policy and Research* (Article Reprint). Washington, D.C. 421-451.

Valle, R. Cultural and Ethnics. In Light, E. & Lebowitz, B. D. (1989). Alzheimer's disease treatment and family stress: directions for research. *U.S. Department of Health and Human Services: Alcohol, Drug Abuse, and Mental Health Administration; National Institute of Mental Health,* 122-154.

Wallace, S.P. & Lew-Ting, C. (1992). Getting by at home–community-based long-term care of latino elders, in cross-cultural medicine–a decade later [Special Issue]. *Western Journal of Medicine 157:*337-344.

Wells, K.B., Golding, J.M., Hough, R.L., Burnam, M.A. & Karno, M. (1988). Factors affecting the probability of use of general and medical health and social/community services for Mexican Americans and non-Hispanic whites. *Medical Care, 26*(5):441-451.

Younoszai, B. (1993). Mexican American perspectives related to death. In Irish, D.P., Lundquist, K.F. & Nelsen, V.J. (eds). *Ethnic Variations in Dying, Death, and Grief.* Washington, D.C.: Taylor and Francis.

Childhood Bereavement Among Cambodians: Cultural Considerations

Linda Lee Prong

SUMMARY. For many children bereavement services are not available until they develop extreme symptoms of chronic grief, post-traumatic stress disorder or depression, if then. This is especially true in some ethnic/racial communities where language and cultural barriers exist. The author uses a review of the literature and interviews with service providers and religious leaders in the Cambodian community of Long Beach to explore those unique cultural factors that have an impact on healthy childhood grief resolution among Cambodian children. Some suggestions for service provision are offered. *[Single or multiple copies of this article are available from The Haworth Document Delivery Service: 1-800-342-9678, 9:00 a.m. - 5:00 p.m. (EST).]*

INTRODUCTION

Helping children cope with childhood bereavement under any circumstances is a difficult task. Typical barriers include: (1) limited funding for

Linda Lee Prong, ACSW, LCSW, is Bereavement Coordinator for Pathways Volunteer Hospice, Adjunct Professor at California State University Long Beach, and a doctoral student in the School of Social Welfare at the University of California Los Angeles.

Address correspondence to: Linda Lee Prong, ACSW, LCSW, Pathways Volunteer Hospice, 3325 Palo Verde Ave., Suite 205, Long Beach, CA 90808.

[Haworth co-indexing entry note]: "Childhood Bereavement Among Cambodians: Cultural Considerations." Prong, Linda Lee. Co-published simultaneously in *The Hospice Journal* (The Haworth Press, Inc.) Vol. 10, No. 2, 1995, pp. 51-64; and: *Hospice Care and Cultural Diversity* (ed: Donna Lind Infeld, Audrey K. Gordon, and Bernice Catherine Harper) The Haworth Press, Inc., 1995, pp. 51-64. Single or multiple copies of this article are available from The Haworth Document Delivery Service: [1-800-342-9678, 9:00 a.m. - 5:00 p.m. (EST)].

children's bereavement services, (2) the lack of exposure children in this country have to death and dying, (3) children's limited ability to verbalize pain and confusion, (4) our limited knowledge of childhood bereavement, and (5) the dearth of intervention research on childhood bereavement. These barriers have resulted in severe restrictions of services to many children until they develop extreme symptoms of chronic grief, post-traumatic stress disorder, or depression. When this situation is further complicated, as it is in the Cambodian community in the United States, by language barriers, cultural differences, multiple losses, and the trauma of war in their native country, assisting bereaved children may become such a formidable task for the hospice provider that the project is abandoned altogether. Understanding those aspects of a culture that present barriers to non-ethnic service providers is essential to develop bereavement programs if the programs are to support ethnic communities in culturally-sensitive ways.

This paper will explore those unique cultural factors in the Cambodian Community in Long Beach, California that have an impact on two prerequisites for healthy childhood grief resolution; clear and open communication about the parent's death and availability of a consistent caregiver in a stable environment. Having previously developed a successful children's bereavement program serving Caucasian, African-American, Hispanic, and some Asian children in the Lakewood/Long Beach community, the Cambodian community presented an exceptional challenge. In order to understand the special needs of this community, besides reviewing the literature, I conducted a series of interviews of service providers and religious leaders involved in the Long Beach Cambodian community. Each service provider was asked for information about the services they provided and the gaps they encountered in service provision. They were also asked to share their understanding of the way the Long Beach Cambodian community approached the issues of death and dying especially as they related to informing or educating children. Where possible, papers or research conducted by the respondents were secured. As information was gathered, it was cross checked with other service providers and the available literature.

THE CAMBODIAN POPULATION IN LONG BEACH

There are an estimated 40,000-60,000 Cambodians residing in Long Beach, California. Representing 10 to 15 percent of the city's population it is the largest concentration of Cambodians outside of Kampuchea (as Cambodia is now called) and refugee camps (Lew, 1990).

Most Cambodians came to this area in the 1980s. They have survived the "Killing Fields" holocaust of the Pol Pot regime during which between 2-3 million Cambodians, one third to half of the population, were killed. Seeing family members tortured, raped, and executed was a common experience for adults and children. Many also endured the trauma of prolonged refugee camp stays where there were additional deaths from disease and malnutrition. For some, the boat trip to this country brought more tragedy, more starvation, drowning incidents, and pirate attacks involving rape and murder.

The younger people, strong enough to withstand such hardships, were those who most often reached safer ports. As a result the U.S. Cambodian population tends to be young. Only 10 percent of the population is 55 or older (Lew, 1990). According to the U.S. Department of Health and Human Services, 21 percent of Cambodians who arrived in this country in 1986 were children 5 and under, many born in refugee camps (Gibbs & Huang, 1989).

Besides personal tragedy, the reign of the Khmer Rouge resulted in the deliberate elimination of elements of Cambodian culture and learning that would normally provide support to grieving families. The educated and intelligentsia were systematically eradicated. Buddhism, the predominant religion of the Cambodian people and a keystone of Cambodian culture, was viewed by the Khmer Rouge as a possible rallying point for opposition forces. Monasteries and Buddhist libraries were destroyed, monks derobed or executed, and traditional ceremonies, including funeral and cremation practices, were prohibited (Sam, 1987).

MITIGATING FACTORS IN THE HEALTHY RESOLUTION OF CHILDHOOD GRIEF FOR CAMBODIAN CHILDREN

Older Cambodian children, as refugees, have a special history of death-related losses not typical of most other children in this country. Many have lost entire families. Although some do not have a conscious memory of Cambodia or the refugee camps, symptoms of post-traumatic stress disorder including unexplained fears, recurrent nightmares, and emotional numbing, as well as adult response to such traumatic losses, may complicate childhood bereavement (Gibbs & Huang, 1989).

Although not personally having experienced the horrors of the Cambodian holocaust, Cambodian children born in this country feel the impact of their family's history. Parents, older siblings, and other adult caregivers may be suffering emotional and somatic symptoms related to previous events that impair their ability to adequately attend to the emotional needs of a grieving child.

Kaffman, Elizur and Gluckson's study (1987) on the impact of a father's death on Israeli children during the war of October 1973 revealed evidence of "pathological disturbance" in children not only in the early months of bereavement but even at 18 and 42 month intervals. This was despite the fact that the children had not witnessed the death, had adequate support systems, suffered no financial strain, and had incurred no other major changes in their lives during this period. The authors identified two pretraumatic factors that appeared to be predictive of a child's initial emotional reaction to the loss: (1) emotional status before the loss, and (2) prolonged separation from one parent before the death. Given the history of the Cambodian refugees it is not surprising to see symptoms–sometimes long standing symptoms–of chronic grief, depression, and post-traumatic stress disorder.

The bereavement literature (Siegel et al., 1990; Kaffman, Elizur et al., 1987) has consistently indicated there are two broadly defined primary conditions that correlate with a child's healthy adjustment to bereavement: (1) clear and open communication about the death of the family member and, (2) a consistent stable environment that includes an available caregiver after the parental death. We will examine these variables in the light of relevant Cambodian cultural factors.

Clear and Open Communication

In a study of a family intervention encouraging parent/child communication after the death of a child's parent, Black and Urbanowicz (1987) found that during the first year of bereavement favorable outcomes in children were heavily associated with the child's ability to cry and talk about the lost parent. This finding is consistent with several other reports (Bowlby, 1969; Brice, 1982; Furman, 1974, 1983; Kaffman et al., 1987; Miller, 1971; Nagera, 1970). This process tends to be suppressed when the surviving parent or caregiver is depressed or unable to respond to the needs of the child for communication about his or her loss. Two years following the loss of the parent this finding regarding communication tends to diminish. Children who have found replacements for the dead parent tend to talk about the deceased less frequently, but this does not seem to presage negative outcomes for children if they have been encouraged to communicate their grief earlier (Black & Urbanowicz, 1987).

Caregiver Availability and Environmental Stability

A second prerequisite for the healthy resolution of childhood grief is a consistent and stable environment that includes at minimum the presence of one caring, available adult. The death of a parent intensifies a child's feelings of vulnerability as well as the lack of control of vital aspects of his or her existence.

While the necessity for meeting basic survival needs is the bottom line, children also have increased needs for love, support, comfort, and reassurance following the death of a parent. A stable, loving parent who is available to provide continuous care is most predictive of positive outcomes for children who have lost a parent (Black & Urbanowicz, 1987; Bowlby, 1980, Garmezy, 1983; Kaffman et al., 1987).

CULTURAL INFLUENCES ON MITIGATING FACTORS

There are four primary cultural factors in the Cambodian community that affect clear and open communication and caregiver availability/environmental stability in major ways: (1) religious beliefs related to the discussion of death and dying, (2) cultural beliefs about the child's role in the family, (3) educational levels and values, and (4) the physical and emotional availability of caregivers. We will examine each of these.

Religious Beliefs Affecting the Discussion of Death and Dying

Religions throughout history have been central to helping families accept, understand, adjust, and give meaning to death and dying. Even though a family may not formally adopt a religion, they will be influenced by the cultural traditions, beliefs, and practices related to death and dying that have evolved in their particular culture under the influence of one or a combination of religions.

The religious beliefs affecting the discussion of death and dying among Cambodians residing in the United States are diverse. Although it must be understood that such beliefs have been influenced by recent events in Kampuchea, and by exposure to western culture, examining the basic religious tenets involved is essential to understanding Cambodian attitudes toward the discussion of death and dying.

While nearly 80 percent of Cambodians still claim to be solidly Buddhist, Khmer Buddhism as practiced in Cambodia is most accurately understood as a combination of Theravada Buddhism, the most clearly delineated element, local animistic folk beliefs, and Brahmanism (Sam, 1987). The way in which Khmer Buddhism is practiced by any given individual will be largely dependent on the degree to which he or she believes and adheres to its various elements.

In addition, exposure to Christianity in the United States, especially the practices of sponsors, has presented another ingredient to the mix. For those who have come over from Cambodia adopting Christianity generally means incorporating it into their existing belief system rather than the total conversion sometimes assumed. Children, on the other hand, may be more open to adopting the major religion of the dominant culture in the absence of the universal reinforcement of Buddhism which existed in Kampuchea.

Theravada Buddhism

Buddhism, as observed by the Cambodian people, was considered a way of life. Often centered around the local monastery, Theravada Buddhism helped people understand the meaning of life and suffering and provided guidelines for dealing with life, suffering, and death. Theravada Buddhism begins with the concept that life is constantly changing. A living being is born, lives through a process of change always becoming something other than it is, dies, and is then reborn through reincarnation. This process of change creates anxiety and pain in the individual who becomes attached to certain people and circumstances in life. The desire to retain that which makes one comfortable and happy creates suffering as it is constantly being thwarted by the reality of a changing existence (Lester, 1973).

The focus of the Theravada Buddhist teaching then is on taking up a path allowing one to deal with the inevitability of suffering (Boehnlein, 1987; Lester, 1973). Change cannot be stopped. Suffering, although inevitable, is not desirable. One's karma or destiny cannot be altered. The only part of the process that can be influenced by the individual is dealing with the desire that creates the suffering. To eliminate the desires is to eliminate the suffering.

Such a philosophy places the responsibility for the suffering squarely on the sufferer. Modification of desire is recommended as an eight-fold path of right living through which the preferred outcome of neither happiness nor pain, but rather a passive acceptance of life, is achieved. One gives no pain and one feels no pain. Not being caught up in emotions allows the individual to concentrate on the pursuit of wisdom and the knowledge of reality.

At first glance, the Buddhist treatment of death would appear to be one of thorough denial. What must be understood is that although apparent emotional passivity is encouraged, a whole series of rituals are performed that allow family members to express feelings symbolically. Veasna Ek described the death of his grandfather in Cambodia. He explained how an entire year was taken up in preparations for the cremation ceremony for this important personage. The body was kept at the local monastery while the family prepared for a huge gathering of friends, neighbors, and well wishers from the village and from other districts. He bemoaned the recent disappearance of such elaborate practices that has allowed families to express their feelings for the deceased in a culturally consistent manner.

Frequently even the most simple ceremonies cannot be practiced by Cambodians in this country. Traditionally, either the "Achaa," who presides over funeral ceremonies, or a Buddhist monk would come and say prayers over the deceased in the family home. The deceased's children would then bathe the corpse and dress it in white (Boehnlein, 1987). The body would then be removed to the Buddhist monastery for still other ceremonies. Since many people in the United States do not die at home, and since corpses are not allowed to be kept in the Buddhist temples here, these traditional practices cannot be adhered to (C. Kong, personal communication, November 18, 1991). Even the traditional pipes, used only for funerals, are seldom used due to the lack of instruments and persons who can play them (V. Ek, personal communication, November 15, 1991).

The focus on passivity in the face of suffering and pain, and the absence of the ceremonies which traditionally provided a vehicle for the expression of grief, clearly mitigates against the open discussion of feelings of grief and pain of bereavement. Families anxious to maintain their Buddhist culture are further reminded of their losses by their inability to celebrate the traditional funeral rites of their culture. While trying to maintain passivity in the face of the loss, they are deprived of the vehicles that provided a means of culturally acceptable and psychologically necessary mourning for the deceased.

Animistic Folk Beliefs

Providing a counterbalance to the Buddhist philosophy of karma, local animistic folk beliefs provided the believer with a sense that his fate might be controlled or influenced by her- or himself. Illness, suffering, and bad luck are thought to come from a variety of spirits when they are offended. Since there are rituals to pacify these spirits, or to avoid offending them in the first place, the spiritual adherent has some influence on the negative circumstances in his or her life. As many of these spirits were specifically related to the dying process, folk beliefs have had a tremendous influence on the grieving practices of the Cambodian community.

Although offering a potential for comfort, folk beliefs have also had some negative implications for adult/child communication during bereavement. Speaking of death is considered unlucky–discussing death is tantamount to inviting it. It is particularly important not to discuss death in front of a person who is injured or ill, and there is also a sense that discussing the subject also will anger the spirits and invite illness, accident, and death (L. Lew, personal communication, November 8, 1991).

Christianity

Christianity is perceived by Cambodians as the dominant religion in the United States. Many refugees' first exposure to Christianity in this country was through sponsors who helped bring them here and who supported their initial attempts at resettlement and adjustment. Accepting Christianity was seen by many Cambodians as both a means of demonstrating appreciation to their sponsors and of becoming Americanized. It should be understood, however, that for most "Christianized" Cambodians, conversion has meant incorporating Christian beliefs, particularly those consistent with pre-existing beliefs, into the current belief systems.

CULTURAL BELIEFS ABOUT THE ROLE OF THE CHILD IN THE FAMILY

Apart from directly affecting the nature of the Cambodian family's bereavement communication, the predominance of Buddhism in Cambodia indirectly contributes to the stability of a child's environment.

Cambodian Family Structure

Cambodia is a largely agrarian society in which the patriarchal family structure was somewhat modified by the Theravada Buddhist emphasis on the individual's need to respect the sanctity of all life through the demonstration of gentleness and tolerance. While the extended family was honored, the respect for all life created far more emphasis on the individual and the couple relationship than typically occurs in Asian countries. Individuals were obligated not only to the society but to find their own path in relation to Buddhist teachings.

Children are highly valued in the Cambodian community. Even children with physical or mental handicaps are cherished although treated in a very paternalistic fashion (L. Lew, personal communication, November 8, 1991). Children are generally expected to be obedient and to respect their parents, helping with family responsibilities as they are able. The Buddhist belief in the inevitability of suffering and the need for discipline to achieve the right thinking and living that bring about spiritual progress reinforces parental expectations and the application of mild physical punishment to achieve these ends.

Adult/Child Communication

The traditional demands for respect and obedience from children promote an atmosphere in which children are not encouraged to talk to adults about personal concerns and emotions. Although a child may get a response to her or his question the first time, further queries are likely to be squelched (V. Ek, personal communication, November 15, 1991). The primacy of the adult role reinforces this stance particularly when the child's need for communication creates discomfort or/and pain for the adult.

One of the tasks of a competent parent is to protect children from experiences perceived as too painful for them to handle. Young children especially, therefore, may not be provided with the information they need to process grief. Even when they ask direct questions children may not be told the truth in order to protect them from "unnecessary" suffering (L. Lew, personal communication, November 8, 1991). Parents often fear nightmares and the spirits that accompany them will cause permanent damage to the child. There is also a fear that young children may offend the spirits of the dead unintentionally by talking with insufficient respect about someone who has died. It is believed that children are less likely to offend potentially harmful spirits if they have less information and do not draw attention to themselves by talking about someone who has died (B. Chittapalo, personal communication, November 18, 1991). Since the spirits are considered to be able to bring illness, mental illness, and even death on the child, such protection is essential.

EDUCATIONAL FACTORS

Educational factors influence the willingness of adult caregivers to provide bereavement support to their children in two major ways. First, the relatively low exposure to formal education among most Cambodians creates a limited understanding of the value of bereavement support and the strategies necessary for obtaining information. Cambodian refugees arriving in this country, on the average, have a fourth grade education (Lew, 1990). The literacy rate in Kampuchea is only about 40 percent (Harkavy, 1991). Service providers find themselves having to work very hard to help parents understand they must support their children's efforts to obtain an education (C. Kong, personal communication, November 18, 1992).

Given these circumstances, it can be easily understood that obtaining information about a subject like childhood bereavement and communicating such information to their children is a low priority for most Cambodian parents. Bereavement educational tools for children do not exist in Cambodian and many adults would not have the literacy skills in either Cambodian or English to take advantage of them, even if they did.

The second result of the lack of education of many adult Cambodians is low exposure to and poor knowledge of mental health practices and services. Although there are indications that Cambodians will make use of mental health services, these are most often accessed in response to somatic complaints, substance abuse, or severe behavioral problems at school. Many Cambodians simply have never learned about the importance of expressing feelings either verbally or nonverbally. Since feeling expression also runs counter to their culture, they can see little value in educating themselves about Western mental health practices.

AVAILABILITY OF CAREGIVERS

The continuity and stability of a child's environment following the death of a parent depends on many factors. As stated previously, most important is the presence of a caring adult who will be consistently available to meet a child's needs. This means that first of all there must be such a person. That person must then be physically and emotionally available to the child. The obstacles present in the current situation of many Cambodian families have precluded such availability.

Physical Availability

For many Cambodian families, parenting figures are lacking because they died in Cambodia, refugee camps, or in the course of emigration. Fifty percent of refugees lost at least one family member before their arrival in refugee camps in Thailand (Oberdorfer, 1987). Extended family members, especially the elderly such as grandparents, who may previously have been available to assume child care, may not be available to Cambodian refugees in this country. Thus, older siblings, aunts, uncles, and cousins frequently accept the responsibility for caring for younger kin (V. Ek, personal communication, November 15, 1991).

Even when caregivers are alive and in the United States they may not be physically available to children. This is true of many because of employment conditions. Cambodians in Long Beach came primarily from rural areas where education was often limited. Their lack of English and industrial job skills forced many into low paying manual labor and service industry positions. Those able to buy their own shops work very long hours. Even when there are two adults in the home they may work alternate shifts to allow one adult to be present when the children are home, even if this parent is asleep. A parent may work a twelve or fourteen hour day leaving little time to give to a child (C. Kong, personal communication, November 18, 1991).

Emotional Availability

When a parent dies, the burden on the family intensifies. A single parent, involved in his or her own grief, struggling to support a family, with limited English and work skills, may be so focused on physical and emotional survival that providing emotional support for a grieving child may have very low priority.

For many Cambodian children the problem of having an "available" adult is not solved by the simple physical presence of a caregiver. The heavy losses experienced by the Cambodian community discussed earlier have resulted in a great deal of depression, chronic grief, and post-traumatic stress disorder in adults. Chow et al. (1989), in a study of Cambodians seen at a non-profit community-based health clinic, found that 65 percent had positive depression scores and 56 percent had positive anxiety scores. Still struggling with nightmares, flashbacks, and other somatic complaints resulting from earlier losses, the discussion of still another loss opens old wounds, renews past losses, and becomes just too painful and difficult to manage especially without supportive mental health services.

RECOMMENDATIONS

Given the limitations of the present situation in the Cambodian community it would seem obvious that hospices wishing to provide bereavement services for these children must be aware of multiple cultural factors. Supportive services must seek to accommodate the current difficult situation of Cambodian refugees rather than offering services which increase demands on already overburdened families.

Since the bereavement literature clearly supports work with parents as the most promising approach for children, hospices will have to be innovative in their programming. While few efforts at collaborating with other agencies have been attempted, this would seem to be the most promising approach in meeting Cambodian children's bereavement needs. Adding a bereavement component to an already existing service program for Cambodians would be one way of maximizing limited culturally sensitive resources. Two programs in Long Beach were open to such collaboration. One is a parenting program, a joint project of the United Cambodian

Community, Inc. and the St. Mary Medical Center, sponsored by the Southeast Asian Health Project, that goes into apartment complexes where Cambodian families are concentrated. The program's Director was very responsive to exploring the addition of a component which would address issues of childhood bereavement, provided by a trained hospice volunteer. A second program, the Long Beach Asian Pacific Mental Health Program, provides limited mental health services to children and was also interested in a collaborative effort to provide services to children even if they were not experiencing severe behavioral problems. One of the greatest advantages in working with existing projects is that they have bilingual staff willing to assist with service delivery and they are already heavily involved in educating adult refugees about the physical and emotional needs of their children in culturally relevant ways.

While the above options may be the best for helping Cambodian children in the long run, other types of collaboration are also possible. Schools particularly have access to children who could be provided with services. Bereavement support groups may be offered in the schools. Usually such groups will have to include Cambodian or Southeastern Asian children with other children unless the school has a particularly large concentration of these children with recent death experiences. Teacher and counselor training using hospice personnel in conjunction with a Cambodian professional who could explain some of the cultural aspects of death and dying might also be useful. While this is not ideal in that it circumvents the parent who needs to be involved in supporting the child, it may be preferable to nothing if other types of collaboration and access are not available.

Cambodians reportedly are more open to using mental health services than other Asian groups (Gibbs & Huang, 1989) and they use these services when they are made available in practical ways (C. Kong, personal communication, November 18, 1992). They show ample evidence of needing the expertise that hospice bereavement programs have developed. Now its up to hospice providers to create culturally relevant services and strategies to reach into the community.

AUTHOR NOTE

This paper would not have been possible without the assistance of several individuals who are already providing a wide variety of services to the Cambodian community in Long Beach. Lillian Lew, Project Director for the Southeast Asian Health Project of the United Cambodian Community, Inc., in conjunction with St. Mary Medical Center, provided introductions to many other service providers and shared her wealth of experience in providing services to the Cambodian Community of Long Beach. Veasna Ek, RN, as the Cambodian Community Worker for the Southeast Asian Health Project, shared his personal story as a Cambodian refugee and teacher in the Thai prison camps and provided valuable information about the Cambodian community as it functions in Long Beach. Rev. Chhean Kong, PhD, who is also Cambodian, is both a clinical psychologist for the Long Beach Asian Pacific Mental Health Program of the Los Angeles County Department of Mental Health and a Buddhist monk. The author is grateful for his having shared his research on the Cambodian community in Long Beach and his insights into the current situation. Bibi Chittapalo spent much time with the author helping her understand the problems of Cambodian children in Long Beach. She is the Cambodian Community worker for the Long Beach Asian Pacific Mental Health Program of the Los Angeles County Department of Mental Health.

The author is grateful to Dr. Cecily Betz, RN, PhD, for advice in the preparation of this manuscript.

REFERENCES

Black, D., & Urbanowicz, M. A. (1987). Family intervention with bereaved children. *Journal of Child Psychology and Psychiatry, 28*(3), 467-476.

Boehnlein, J. K. (1987). Clinical relevance of grief and mourning among Cambodian refugees. *Social Science and Medicine, 25*(7), 765-772.

Bowlby, J. (1969). *Attachment and Loss. Vol 1*. London: Hogarth Press.

Bowlby, J. (1980). *Loss*. New York: Basic Books.

Brice, C. W. (1982). Mourning throughout the life cycle. *The American Journal of Psychoanalytic Association, 11*, 500-541.

Chow, R. T., Krumholtz, S., & Landau, C. (1989). Psychological screening of Cambodian refugees in a RI primary care clinic. *Rhode Island Medical Journal, 72*, 279-281.

Furman, E. (1974). *A child's parent dies*. New Haven: Yale University Press.

Furman, E. (1983). Studies in childhood bereavement. *Canadian Journal of Psychiatry, 28* (4) 241-247.

Garmezy, N. (1983). Stressors of Childhood, In N. Garmezy & M. Rutter (Eds.) *Stress, Coping and Development in Children*. New York: McGraw-Hill.

Gibbs, J. T. & Huang, L. N. (Eds.) (1989). *Children of color: Psychological interventions with minority youth*. San Francisco: Jossey-Bass Publishers, (278-321).

Goodyer, I. M. (1990). Family relationships, life events and childhood psychopathology. *Journal of Child Psychology and Psychiatry, 31*(1), 161-192.

Harkavy, M. D. (Ed.) (1991). *The American spectrum encyclopedia*. New York: American Booksellers Association, (587-588).

Kaffman, M., Elizur, E., & Gluckson, L. (1987). Bereavement reactions in children: Therapeutic implications. *1st Journal of Psychiatry and Related Sciences, 24*(1-2), 65-76.

Lester, R. C. (1973). *Theravada Buddhism in Southeast Asia*. Ann Arbor, MI: The University of Michigan Press.

Lew, L. (1990). *Elderly Cambodians in Long Beach: Creating Cultural access to health care*. Unpublished manuscript.

Miller, J. B. (1971). Children's reactions to the death of a parent. *Journal of the American Psychoanalytic Association, 19*, 697-719.

Nagera, H. (1970). Children's reactions to the death of important objects: A developmental approach. *Psychoanalytic Study of the Child, 25*, 360-400.

Oberdorfer, D. (1987, March 3). Indochinese Americans seek help for refugees. *Washington Post*, A18.

Sam, Y. (1987). *Khmer Buddhism and politics from 1954 to 1984*. Newington, CT: Khmer Studies Institute.

Siegal, K., Mesagno, F. P., Christ, G. (1990). A prevention program for bereaved children. *American Journal of Orthopsychiatry, 60*(2) 168-175.

Deterrents to Access and Service for Blacks and Hispanics: The Medicare Hospice Benefit, Healthcare Utilization, and Cultural Barriers

Audrey K. Gordon

SUMMARY. The Medicare Hospice Benefit may limit access for Blacks and Hispanics because of its requirement of continuity of care, entailing the availability of a primary caregiver. The literature on utilization of healthcare services by Blacks and Hispanics shows these groups were likely to receive too little care, too late. Kalish and Reynolds' (1976) research on attitudes of Blacks, Mexican-Americans, and Whites toward dying shows cultural differences that could affect acceptance of hospice philosophy. In other research reviewed in this paper distrust of White service providers was a significant cultural barrier for Blacks in using health services. Lack of familiarity with the health care system and language barriers were barriers most often for Hispanics. Black caregivers are more likely than Whites to have dying persons living with them, to be extended family members or nonrelated, and to be more limited in their ability to provide caregiving support because of a lack of economic resources. Hispanics appear to have a circumscribed support system,

Audrey K. Gordon, PhD, is Assistant Professor and Senior Researcher at the University of Illinois at Chicago, School of Public Health.

Address correspondence to: Audrey K. Gordon, PhD, University of Illinois at Chicago, School of Public Health, 2121 W. Taylor, Rm. 217, Chicago, IL 60612.

[Haworth co-indexing entry note]: "Deterrents to Access and Service for Blacks and Hispanics: The Medicare Hospice Benefit, Healthcare Utilization, and Cultural Barriers." Gordon, Audrey K. Co-published simultaneously in *The Hospice Journal* (The Haworth Press, Inc.) Vol. 10, No. 2, 1995, pp. 65-83; and: *Hospice Care and Cultural Diversity* (ed: Donna Lind Infeld, Audrey K. Gordon, and Bernice Catherine Harper) The Haworth Press, Inc., 1995, pp. 65-83. Single or multiple copies of this article are available from The Haworth Document Delivery Service: [1-800-342-9678, 9:00 a.m. - 5:00 p.m. (EST)].

narrowly defined by blood kinship, with females as the expected caregivers. *[Single or multiple copies of this article are available from The Haworth Document Delivery Service: 1-800-342-9678, 9:00 a.m. - 5:00 p.m. (EST).]*

INTRODUCTION

Now that hospice is firmly entrenched as part of the Medicare system, a closer examination of the issues that might affect minority utilization of hospice care is warranted. Some charge the U.S. healthcare system lacks adequate services for the poor and uninsured, has inequities in the distribution and quality of services, lacks minority professionals, and is indifferent to culturally-sensitive issues that affect on access and delivery of services to diverse racial/ethnic groups (Davis, 1985; Davis and Rowland, 1983; Heckler, 1985; Strauss and Corbin, 1988). Availability of continuity of care and a primary caregiver in a stable home environment, often criteria for hospice admission, may make use of hospice care by culturally diverse groups more difficult. Black and Hispanic cultural values about healthcare and dying may require understanding and modification of hospice practice in order to attract patients and families. Early discussions of the Medicare regulations suggested that the regulations described patients and families from the mainstream of America and created barriers for disadvantaged groups.

EARLY CRITICISMS OF THE MEDICARE
HOSPICE REGULATIONS

The Medicare Hospice Benefit (MHB), the only human service legislation of the Reagan Congress, passed into law in November 1983. Although hailed as a triumph for hospice by making federal reimbursement available, it soon became clear that its requirements imposed a new set of constraints on hospice admissions. Most of the literature between 1983-1988 discusses the initiation of the MHB and its effect on hospice, especially concerning patient admissions and doctor/hospital relationships with hospice organizations (Abel, 1986; Amenta, 1984; Greer et al., 1988; Mor, 1987a; Paradis, 1984; Torrens, 1985).

Criticisms of the regulations consistently recognized that access to the benefit was limited by financial incentives to enroll patients with a particular kind of profile. The preferred patient was middle-class, married and living with a spouse at home, and with the type of cancer that presents as a rapid-growing solid tumor with few other complications (Abel, 1986; Amenta, 1984; Fraser, 1985; Kusserow, 1984). Patients for whom the strongest financial disincentives applied lived alone, were dying from diseases with indefinite prognoses, had complications from the disease process requiring frequent inpatient stays, had little or no family support available for care in the home, lived at a distance from the nearest hospice, and might be predisposed by culture or personality not to talk about impending death (Abel, 1986; Amenta, 1984; Amenta, 1985; Mor et al., 1989; Fraser, 1985; Kusserow, 1984; Martin, 1984).

Abel recognized that "the [MHB] emphases on home care discriminated against hospices located in inner urban areas, where a high proportion of the population lives alone," and she noted that hospices were "disproportionately in suburban communities" (Abel, 1986). Mor found hospice patients who were unable to be cared for at home tended to have less social support, be more functionally deteriorated, have working caregivers, and less supportive family systems (Mor et al., 1988). This profile is consistent with Kane's description of hospice patients in a Veterans Administration hospital (VA) and Torrens' description of hospice patients served by the VA. Torrens also points out that frequently it is minority patients who fit this profile (Kane, 1984; Torrens, 1985).

The MHB 80/20 rule may have influenced which model of hospice could profitably become certified and what kind of patient was excluded from hospice services. The 80/20 payment rule is a cost containment strategy limiting reimbursement to a maximum of 20% of the total annual Medicare reimbursement at the acute care per diem rate with 80% reimbursement for lower rates. Since the Brown University demonstration identified the hospital-based hospice as providing 29% of patient care on the inpatient unit, and showed that hospital-based care was more costly than care delivered by the community-based model (Amenta, 1985; Mor, 1987a), the MHB curtailed utilization of acute care. Thus the home or residential nursing facility became the preferred site of care (Lynn, 1985; Greer et al., 1988). Because of the 80/20 rule, the hospital-based hospice inpatient unit incurred the possibility of greater financial risk in serving patients, often without family support and with complicated needs, who required extended inpatient stays (Mor, 1987a).

The MHB regulation also required core services. If a hospital could not provide nursing and other core services to the home, it could not become Medicare certified as a hospice. Chicago is a good example of an urban area with underserved minorities. In Chicago, the hospitals that do not deliver home health services are public or teaching hospitals serving large numbers of poor and minorities. As of 1994, in inner-city Chicago, hospitals that do not have their own home health programs include Cook County Hospital, the University of Illinois Hospital, Michael Reese Hospital, and the University of Chicago Hospitals. These four teaching hospitals together serve more poor and minorities than other hospitals in the city. Each of these hospitals, except Cook County, has a contract with independent or home health agency-based hospices but do not offer hospital-owned hospice services to patients. Cook County Hospital offers a palliative care service in an inpatient unit restricted to patients referred by staff physicians and may refer patients to other hospices.

Thus the legislation provided disincentives for hospitals to certify for the benefit (Amenta, 1985; Amenta, 1984; Martin, 1984; Mor et al., 1988). Hospitals responded either by giving up their hospice unit, maintaining it as a community service and absorbing the cost, or contracting for beds with community-based hospices. Only when hospitals began diversifying into the growing market of home care services about 1987 did they begin to certify for the benefit. Hospice units in Veterans Administration hospitals did not experience these problems since their patients are insured by CHAMPUS, not Medicare.

The legislation that established a reimbursement cap for each patient also influenced or restricted hospice access because, unlike other parts of Medicare, the cap did not adjust for age, disability, and geographic location. "This puts the hospice at risk for significant variations in patient population, duration of care, and expenditures for different types of cancer" (Martin, 1984). The cap discourages service to heavy-use, difficult-to-serve patients or patients with complicated morbidity.

Pawling-Kaplan and O'Connor (1987) conducted a survey of the entire population of hospices to examine the effect of Medicare certification on the admission requirement for a primary caregiver (PCP). This research tracked the impact of the primary caregiver requirement from 1980 through 1986. "The results of this study suggested that federal regulations may have had an effect on access to hospice care by encouraging admission policy decisions that discriminate against persons who have no available primary caregiver" (Ibid.). According to the Department of Health and Human Services, the primary caregiver is someone available in the home at least nineteen hours per day. Based on this definition "the Medicare guidelines maintain profoundly unrealistic expectations of caregivers" who are frequently unable to remain at home (MacDonald, 1989).

Medicare certification can greatly expand hospice access. Increasing the patient base brings more reimbursement dollars into the budget, allowing the hospice to provide more charitable services or serve more difficult cases (Lee, 1988, personal communication). If a hospice is Medicare certified, it will also be Medicaid certified in states offering Medicaid hospice reimbursement. Where reimbursement exists, hospices with a large patient census can serve more costly patients.

HEALTH BEHAVIORS AFFECTING ACCESS

Knowledge of a service is often a necessary precondition or enabling factor for its use. The Supplement on Aging to the 1984 National Health Interview Survey was analyzed by Mor, Hendershot, and Cryan (1989) for recognition of and familiarity with the hospice concept. Over half (53%) of respondents aged fifty-five or older were unfamiliar with hospice; of those familiar with it, only 48.5% knew where to obtain it. Females of all ages were more likely to know about it than men (Mor et al., 1989; Richman and Rosenfeld, 1988). A strong linear relationship existed between level of education and hospice knowledge. Previous history of association with cancer had less significance than hypothesized (Ibid., 1989).

The pattern of hospice awareness varied by geographic region. This finding may reflect the typical location of hospices in large urban or middle-class suburban areas. Mor concluded that, although education was a strong factor in hospice recognition, the most relevant access issue was probably the awareness of the provider and not consumer awareness (Ibid.).

Physician familiarity with hospice is essential since they most influence the patients' knowledge about and access to hospice care (Bulkin and Lukashok, 1988; Gordon, 1989). A survey conducted annually since 1983 by the Illinois State Hospice Organization (ISHO) shows that the primary referral source to hospice is the physician. Family/friends and hospital discharge planners are second and third respectively (ISHO, 1983-89, unpublished data).

If access to a physician influences access to hospice care, then it may be hypothesized that minorities, who are less likely to have an attending physician than Whites, would be referred less often. Because many minorities are low income and/or uninsured, their health care practices are often determined primarily by their financial status and the medical services available to them (Davis and Rowland, 1983; Strauss and Corbin, 1988). Only those few instances where hospice services are offered as part of a public hospital or health department, such as Grady County Hospital in Atlanta, are hospice services readily available to economically disadvantaged groups (Granger and Moore, 1990).

An important characteristic, then, for hospice access is continuity of care defined as regular and ongoing access to a physician or group of physicians. Continuity of care generally is not found among the poor and minorities. The Report of the Secretary's Task Force on Black and Minority Health (Heckler, 1985) cites the following:

- More Blacks and Hispanics than Whites report that they have no usual source of medical care.
- Fewer Blacks and Hispanics than Whites report that they use a physician's office as their usual source of care.
- Twice as many Blacks and Hispanics than Whites report they use hospital and health clinics as their usual source of medical care.
- More than 25% of all visits made to physicians by Blacks occurred in hospital clinics or emergency rooms compared to 11% by Whites.

Other data on minority health utilization reveal similar findings of lack of access to regular care and an increased population in fair or poor health (Butler, 1988; Davis, 1985). In the 1986 Robert Wood Johnson National Access Survey, Blacks and Hispanics reported fair to poor health, more chronic or serious illness, fewer visits for medical care in the previous year, and were less likely to have a regular source of health care. In addition, Hispanics used emergency rooms more often than Whites or Blacks and were overwhelmingly without health insurance. The report concluded that "The most disturbing findings ... involve the deterioration in access to medical care among the nation's poor, minority, and uninsured citizens" (Leon, 1987).

Utilization of public health hospitals and clinics for ordinary medical care may be a legacy of the southern experience where Blacks were routinely denied access to private providers and received their medical care from public "second class institutions" (Weaver, 1976). Since emergency rooms are available twenty-four hours, seven days a week, Blacks and Hispanics may resort to emergency room use in nonwork hours.

Continuity of care strikes at the very heart of hospice admission criteria: the attending physician must be available to care for the patient. Medicare also requires that *both* the attending physician and the hospice physician document the eligibility of the patient. If there is not an attending physician to make this diagnosis, evaluation for and referral to hospice is much more difficult.

POSSIBLE CULTURAL BARRIERS TO HOSPICE USE
FOR BLACKS AND MEXICAN-AMERICANS

In the 1970s Kalish and Reynolds studied attitudes toward death and dying within four ethnic groups: Whites, Blacks, Japanese-Americans and Mexican-Americans (Kalish and Reynolds, 1976). The 434 respondents were evenly distributed among the four ethnic groups, with sampling controls on median family income. Every census tract in which the median income was above that of Los Angeles County was eliminated. Thus, subjects sampled were from low and middle-income families. The elderly population was oversampled, adding validity to the findings for hospice, since the elderly are the overwhelming majority of hospice patients. Subjects were interviewed in their language of choice.

Although hospice was not available in the U.S. at the time of the study, the answers to certain questions may suggest these groups' attitudes toward hospice philosophy and care (See Figures 1 and 2). Since hospice utilization by Asian-Americans is not a primary focus of this paper, only the results for Blacks, Whites and Mexican-Americans are reported here.

Black Americans had the lowest preference for death at home, preferring undefined "other" sites over the hospital. The definition of other sites is unclear. Blacks also reported the least need to have family mem-

FIGURE 1. Preferred Location for Death

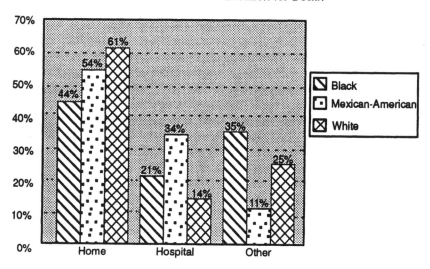

Kalish and Reynolds (1976)

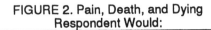

FIGURE 2. Pain, Death, and Dying
Respondent Would:

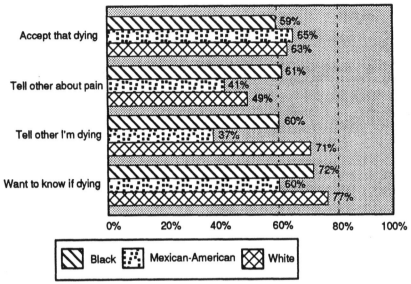

Kalish and Reynolds (1976)

bers spend time with them. This need for family members *decreased* with increasing age as religious belief and the church community replaced the family for social support (Kalish and Reynolds, 1976). Contradictory findings were reported in a later study, where 62% of Blacks surveyed preferred to die in a hospital rather than at home, however, this study did not control for income and age (Neubauer and Hamilton, 1990).

Blacks have been reported to have a high expectation of living a long life which is often founded in religious faith (Kalish & Reynolds, 1976). This expectation could result in a cultural barrier to hospice use. In reality, Blacks experience a shorter life expectancy and increased morbidity and mortality from cancer, strokes, and diabetes (Heckler, 1985).

Mexican-Americans and Whites reported a greater reluctance to admit pain than Blacks. The willingness to tell someone about pain could result in relief-seeking behavior. This is important because the acknowledged presence of pain is a frequent motivator in the initiation of hospice care (Personal communications with hospice directors).

Willingness to admit that someone is dying is also a key criterion in acceptance of hospice services. Hospices, like other medical providers of care, require informed consent. If an ethnic group has a taboo against open communication on this issue, it would be difficult for members of that group to use hospice services without some opprobrium from the community. Nearly three-quarters of all Whites, followed by nearly two-thirds of all Blacks, report they would want someone told they were dying, but only one-third of Mexican-Americans would want someone to know. Such denial could make the philosophy of open communication and the requirement of informed consent cultural barriers for Mexican-Americans in the use of hospice services. Fewer barriers appear to exist in the other groups.

White subjects are more likely to report the characteristics required to accept hospice philosophy: a willingness to be told about impending death and acceptance of prognosis, a preference to die at home, and a willingness to discuss dying with family members. A relatively high percentage of Mexican Americans and Whites were willing to endure pain in silence. Religion may play a part in attitudes toward pain. For White Anglo-Saxon Protestants, expressions of outward suffering are considered undignified. Stoicism and mastery are primary values of the culture. For many Catholics, suffering may be seen as ennobling and God's will and as a test of faith. Another factor may be social class. Disadvantaged groups may have learned to "endure" since their outcries would not have brought them some surcease from pain in the past (Leyhe et al., 1972).

In summary there may be cultural barriers to hospice use in Black and Mexican-American communities based on place of death and communicating with the dying person. All three groups reported similar levels of acceptance of death, the willingness to talk about prognosis, and communication about pain. Therefore these cultural differences require attention but may not be insurmountable obstacles to hospice utilization.

PATTERNS OF HEALTHCARE UTILIZATION AFFECTING ACCESS

The Black Community

Most of what has been written about the use of hospice care by the Black community is very recent. Black leaders have criticized the underutilization of hospice services by Blacks and have attempted to increase participation through education, staffing, and greater cultural sensitivity (Granger and Moore, 1990; Harper, 1990; McDonald, 1990; Meyers, 1990). Lundgren and Chen (1986) cite barriers to hospice use by Blacks as "lack of availability, lack of community awareness, lack of trust of social service providers, and misperceptions of the role of hospice service." The first two barriers, lack of availability and lack of community awareness, could apply to any group, but the last two, lack of trust of social service providers and misperception of the role of hospice services may be factors specific to the Blacks. Lack of trust of social services arises from reliance on a life long kinship network as a major coping mechanism, especially in times of stress. Strangers from hospice, seen as mainstream healthcare providers, may not be welcomed into the intimacy of a racial/ethnic family (Gordon and Rooney, 1984).

The frequent hospice requirement of a primary caregiver (PCP) in the home is a further deterrent. Members of the Black family usually have to work and no one is available for this caregiving role (Lundgren and Chen, 1986). Since many lower income families may have all family members working, the PCP requirement may exclude patients by income status, not race or ethnicity (Lynn, 1985; Pawling-Kaplan and O'Connor, 1989; Rhymes, 1990).

Discomfort with the concept of palliative care in the Black community may be based on the belief that God and personal faith prohibits giving up (Kalish and Reynolds, 1976; Neubauer and Hamilton, 1990). Since hospice is palliative, not curative, and requires recognizing that death is near and unavoidable, its use could be seen as not fighting to live. Lundgren and Chen conclude that ways of working within the multigenerational extended family and the church must be developed in order for hospice to succeed in the Black community (Lundgren and Chen, 1986).

The Hispanic Community

One theory of Mexican-American health care behavior posits four basic sources of health care knowledge and treatment: (1) folk medical lore of medieval Spain as refined in Mexico, (2) one or more native American tribes, (3) Anglo [White] folk medicine, and (4) scientific medicine. Folk medicine is based on health as a matter of chance; Magic and bewitchment cause many illnesses (Weaver, 1976). Falicov (1982) observed that, while nearly all Mexican-Americans are Roman Catholic, "sorcery, witchcraft and ancient herbal lore exist along with Western medical practices and beliefs."

Older studies show that Mexican-Americans have a fatalistic attitude toward illness (Clark, 1959; Rubel, 1960). Rubel identified the fee system of U.S. health care as an irritant to Mexican-Americans since folk healers receive "gratuities" and are seen as helping the people; physicians charging fees are seen as enriching themselves at the expense of the people.

Health care utilization by Mexican-Americans may be underreported. They may be reluctant to approach the medical care system for fear of investigation by authorities (Sotomayor, 1988; Weaver, 1976).

Middle and upper income Mexican-Americans show no significant differences in health care behavior from Whites, other than preferring treatment by Spanish speaking personnel (Solis et al., 1990; Weaver, 1976). The importance of language as a barrier to health care access was revealed in the Hispanic Health and Nutrition Examination Study (HHANES) 1982-84. " . . . [T]he ability to speak English increases the extent to which Hispanics can effectively gain institutional access . . . [and] . . . access is strongly related to utilization" (Solis et al., 1990). Data substantiate that large portions of Hispanics do not have a regular health care provider or health insurance. Further, Mexican-Americans are the most likely of the three Hispanic groups studied to be affected by the access variables of language, financial constraints, geographic inaccessibility, lack of transportation and lack of a regular source of care (Estrada et al., 1990). The HHANES analysis also suggests that Medicaid eligibility criteria may restrict access to health services in some states (Solis et al., 1990). The lack of a Medicaid Hospice Benefit in some states may also play a part in the inability of medically-underserved populations to access hospice care.

Unfortunately, studies of health behavior are often distorted because of lack of controls on social class, age, and education. In addition, studies of Hispanics suffer from inaccurate reporting of health data, lack of cross-sectional sampling, and a lack of varied geographic sampling (Sotomayor and Randolph, 1988a; Sidel and Sidel, 1983; Weaver, 1976). Weaver believes that the stereotypes of Hispanic health behaviors describe lower class Mexican-American behavior because this is the most accessible group for study.

CAREGIVING AND SUPPORT SYSTEMS
FOR BLACKS AND HISPANICS

There is considerable disagreement whether support systems and caregiving roles among Blacks and Hispanics differ from those of Whites, and, when they do differ, whether that difference can be attributed to the culture or to socioeconomic variables (Anderson and Dilworth-Anderson, in press; Chatters et al., 1986; Chevan and Korson, 1972; De La Rosa, 1989; Delgado and Humm-Delgado, 1982; Hanson, 1983; Hill, 1972; Mitchell and Register, 1984; Mutran, 1985).

Studies of caregiving and support systems among Blacks show that the kin network is the primary provider of extensive support to family members, closely followed by informal support from church members used especially at times of illness (Chevan and Korson, 1972; Gelfand, 1982; Gibson and Jackson, 1989; Hays and Mindel, 1973; Hanson et al., 1983; Hill, 1972; Jackson, 1980; Mitchell and Register, 1984; Rubenstein, 1971; Taylor and Chatters, 1986). This network differs from those of Whites and Hispanics in that nonblood kin are considered equal to blood members in terms of status and responsibilities toward family members. This view of family composition is based on a cultural interpretation of the Black family shaped by its uprooting from Africa and its need to recreate an extended family. That accounts for the "strong sense of group solidarity or 'We-ness' in the Black community" (Brown, 1989; Nobles, 1974).

Other researchers contend that the strong Black family support network is a result of economic necessity (Chevan and Korson, 1972; Mutran, 1985) and, when socio-economic factors are controlled, there are few significant differences in caregiving roles and attitudes in Black and White support systems (Anderson and Dilworth-Anderson, in press; Hanson, 1983; Mitchell and Register, 1984). One possible explanation why Black families (and other ethnic groups) are portrayed as having such strong bonds is that ethnic writers tend to use family structure as a symbol of their ethnic values.

In a study pairing volunteers by race, greater help and support were reported by the matched population, controlling for other socio-economic variables. Black volunteers received more support from their community when helping Blacks than they received in White communities when helping Whites (Morrow-Howell et al., 1990). This has implications for hospices in serving any culturally diverse group, especially when using volunteers in the intimacy of the home (Gordon and Rooney, 1984). There is a need, not only for more education about different cultures, but for the recruitment of staff and volunteers from the groups to be served.

Other studies show a high level of mistrust of Whites and White institutions among Blacks (Terrell and Terrell, 1981) and greater probability for noncompliance when using traditional medical care (Anderson and Dilworth-Anderson, in press). Similarly Hispanics avoid healthcare organizations because of culturally insensitive medical practices (Sotomayor and Randolph, 1988b). This noncompliance in and avoidance of health care in part can be attributed to the "culture of medicine" and to a lack of cultural sensitivity. The culture of medicine " . . . is comprised of the particular habits, customs, and expectations of health professionals as well as the needs of the bureaucratic organizations in which they work" (Riessman, 1986). To low income and minority patients this culture may seem " ... terribly massive and complex, crowded and busy; while the personnel seem often impersonal, brusque, or even insulting ... " (Strauss, 1972). The preference for reliance on kinship groups and folk healers at times of illness therefore may be reinforced by the negative experiences of minority groups in health care settings.

Research on Hispanic elderly is limited and little is known about support systems and utilization of health care and human services in Hispanic subpopulation groups. Literature suggests that formal systems are underutilized primarily due to the cultural insensitivities of providers and socioeconomic factors affecting access (e.g., citizenship status or lack of insurance) and to a preference by Hispanics for their own indigenous helping structures and modalities (Sotomayor, 1988).

Other studies suggest Mexicans and Puerto Ricans are more closely involved in reciprocal relationships, primarily with their daughters, than other groups in the majority society. However there is little information on how different Hispanic subgroups use intergenerational networks during time of need (Sotomayor and Randolph, 1988a). In contrast to the Black community where support across three or four generations was common (Anderson and Dilworth-Anderson, in press), a study of Puerto Rican elderly showed reliance on children but not grandchildren (Bastida, 1988). Bastida also suggests that the support of the current child cohort may not be available in the future due to economic factors and the assimilation of younger Hispanics into Western culture. By the year 2000, the Hispanic population over 75 will have grown considerably and will add significant demands to already strained health and human service resources (Sotomayor and Randolph, 1988b).

Other variables cause difficulties in providing support services to Hispanic elderly outside the family system. Mexican-Americans have the second highest illiteracy rate in the U.S. among racial/ethnic groups (Census, 1987) and illiteracy and monolinguality tend to be highest among the elderly. The groups at highest risk for poor health and stress are monolingual Mexican-American women, ages 40-59, and men, ages 60-69 (Curiel and Rosenthal, 1988). The challenge of providing formal health and support services to Mexican-American elderly is greater than provision to Blacks and Whites, even controlling for income. Hispanics prefer using informal kinship groups to formal support systems (Curiel and Rosenthal, 1988; Korte and Villa, 1988). Hispanic families, therefore, tend not to use nursing homes, hospitals, and other specialized agencies.

Anzaldua identified predominant coping styles among low-income Hispanics for stress control as increased religiosity, helplessness, passive acceptance, and resignation (Anzaldua et al., 1988). Less than one-third of the group studied attempted to modify stressful situations by taking direct action, seeking help, or, least of all, mobilizing support. These coping styles may reflect the theology of Hispanic Catholicism in fostering a passive acceptance of life (and death). If passive acceptance (Ibid.) is characteristic of those who need to reach out for medical care and support, then only immediate family members, through personal observation, will be able to identify these needs and it is they who will be called upon to meet them. Some of those caregivers, especially the elderly, are likely to accept situations of terminal illness passively. If, as reported, Hispanic culture does not expect men to be caregivers (Bastida, 1988), then the number of persons available in the caregiving role is severely limited.

CONCLUSION

Limitations to hospice access affect disadvantaged socio-economic groups because of constraints within the Medicare regulations or patterns of healthcare utilization that differ from the mainstream American population. These limitations disproportionately affect Blacks and Hispanics. Continuity of care and requirements for primary caregivers remain stumbling-blocks for low income and minority patients (Beresford, 1995).

While there are cultural differences in the degree of open communication about issues of terminal illness, these differences alone should not impede hospice use. Caregiving patterns vary in Black and Hispanic families and require attention in order to make hospice services minimally intrusive at a time of great stress. Black caregivers (and decision-makers) may not be related to the patient, while Hispanics, favoring informal healthcare networks, expect female family members to provide care. Both groups remain wary of the U.S. healthcare system based on their experiences, with Hispanics especially critical of the lack of bilingual services.

Service to minorities will grow as knowledge about and experiences with hospice increase. Efforts to make culturally diverse groups comfortable and to target the recruitment and training of minority health professionals for hospices would make hospice care "culturally-friendly." Black and Hispanic national and community organizations can be invited to participate in evaluating and changing admission criteria that adversely affect minorities. These organizations can also be enlisted to provide education about hospice to their members. These are some of the ways hospices can meet the challenge of caring for culturally diverse and economically disadvantaged populations.

REFERENCES

Abel, E. (1986). The hospice movement: Institutionalizing innovation. *International Journal of Health Services, 16*(1), 71-83.

Amenta, M. O. (1984). Hospice USA 1984–Steady and holding. *Oncology Nursing Forum, 11*(5), 68-74.

Amenta, M. O. (1985). Hospice in the United States: Multiple models and varied programs. *Nursing Clinics of North America, 20*(2), 269-279.

Anderson, N. B., & Dilworth-Anderson, P. (in press). Dementia caregiving in Blacks: A contextual approach. In E. Light (Ed.), *Family Caregiving and Stress.* New York: Springer Press.

Anzaldua, H., Reed-Sanders, D., Wrinkle, R. D., & Gibson, G. (1988). Coping styles of Mexican American elderly. In M. Sotomayor, & H. Curiel (Eds.), *Hispanic Elderly: A Cultural Signature* (pp. 95-116). Edinburg: Pan American University Press.

Bastida, E. (1988). Reexamining traditional assumptions about extended familism: Older Puerto Ricans in a comparative perspective. In M. Sotomayor, & H. Curiel (Eds.), *Hispanic Elderly: A Cultural Signature* (pp. 163-184). Edinburg: Pan American University Press.

Beresford, L. (1995, Winter). Home alone: The challenge of caring for patients without caregivers. *Hospice,* 21-24.

Brown, N. (1989). Afro-Caribbean spirituality: A Haitian case study. *Second Opinion, 11*(July), 36-57.

Bulkin, W., & Lukashok, H. (1988). Rx for dying: The case for hospice. *The New England Journal of Medicine, 318*(6), 376-378.

Butler, P. A. (1988). *Too Poor To Be Sick.* Washington, D.C: American Public Health Association.

Chatters, L., Taylor, R., & Jackson, J. (1986). Aged blacks' choice for an informal helper network. *Journal of Gerontology, 41*(1), 94-100.

Chevan, A., & Korson, J. H. (1972). The widowed who live alone: An examination of social and demographic factors. *Social Work, 15,* 45-53.

Clark, M. (1959). *Health in the Mexican-American Culture.* Berkeley: University of California Press.

Curiel, H., & Sotomayor, M. (1988). Future directions and the development of programs for the Hispanic elderly. In M. Sotomayor, & H. Curiel (Eds.), *Hispanic Elderly: A Cultural Signature* (pp. 247-254). Edinburg: Pan American University Press.

Curiel, H., & Rosenthal, J. A. (1988). The influence of aging on self-esteem: A consideration of ethnicity, gender, and acculturation level differences. In M. Sotomayor, & H. Curiel (Eds.), *Hispanic Elderly: A Cultural Signature* (pp. 11-32). Edinburg: Pan American University Press.

Davis, K., & Rowland, D. (1983). Uninsured and underserved: Inequities in health care in the United States. *Milbank Memorial Fund Quarterly/Health and Society, 61*(2), 149-177.

Davis, K. (1985). *Access to health care: A matter of fairness* (17). Washington, D.C.: Center for National Policy.

De La Rosa, M. (1989). Health care needs of Hispanic Americans and the responsiveness of the health care system. *Health and Social Work,* (May), 104-113.

Delgado, M., & Humm-Delgado, D. (1982). Natural support systems: A source of strength in Hispanic communities. *Social Work, 27*(1), 83-89.

Estrada, A. L., Trevino, F. M., & Ray, L. A. (1990). Health care utilization barriers among Mexican-Americans: Evidence from HHANES 1982-84. *American Journal of Public Health, 80*(Supplement), 27-31.

Falicov, C. J. (1982). Mexican families. In M. McGoldrick, J. K. Pearce, & J. Giordano (Eds.), *Ethnicity and Family Therapy* (pp. 134-163). New York: The Guilford Press.

Fraser, I. (1985). Medicare reimbursement for hospice care: Ethical and policy implications of cost-containment strategies. *Journal of Health Politics, Policy and Law, 10*(3), 565-578.

Gelfand, D. (1982). *Aging: The Ethnic Factor.* Boston: Little, Brown and Company.

Gibson, R., & Jackson, J. (1989). The health, physical functioning, and informal supports of the Black elderly. In D. P. Willis (Ed.), *Health Policies and Black Americans* (pp. 421-454). New Brunswick: Transaction Publishers.

Gordon, A. K., & Rooney, A. (1984). Hospice and the family: A systems approach to assessment. *American Journal of Hospice Care, 1*(1), 31-33.

Gordon, A. K. (1989). The physician gatekeeper: Access to the Medicare hospice benefit. *The American Journal of Hospice Care, 6*(5), 44-48.

Granger, V. C., & Moore, M. R. (1990). Marketing and minorities: Hospice in the Black community. *The American Journal of Hospice and Palliative Care, 7*(September/October), 20-26.

Greer, D., Mor, V., & Kastenbaum, R. (1988). Public policy and the hospice movement. In V. Mor, D. Greer, & R. Kastenbaum (Eds.), *The Hospice Experiment* (pp. 227-244). Baltimore: The Johns Hopkins University Press.

Hanson, S., Sauer, W., & Seelbach, W. (1983). Racial and cohort variations in filial responsibility norms. *The Gerontologist, 23*(4), 626-631.

Harper, B. C. (1990, Spring). Doing the right thing: Three strategies for increasing minority involvement. *Hospice,* 14-15.

Hays, W., & Mindel, C. H. (1973). Extended kin relations in Black and White families. *Marriage and the Family, 35,* 51-55.

Heckler, M. (1985). *Report of the Secretary's Task Force on Black and Minority Health* (Vol. 1, Executive Summary). Department of Health and Human Services. Washington, D.C.: U.S. Government Printing Office.

Hill, R. B. (1972). A profile of the Black aged. In Institute of Gerontology (Ed.),

Minority Aged in America (pp. 35-50). Ann Arbor: University of Michigan Press.

Jackson, J. J. (1980). *Minorities and Aging.* Belmont: Wadsworth Publications.

Kalish, R. & Reynolds, D. (1976). *Death and Ethnicity: A Psychocultural Study.* Farmingdale, New York: Baywood Publishing.

Kane, R. L., Wales, J., Bernstein, L., Leibowitz, A., & Kaplan, S. (1984). A randomised controlled trial of hospice care. *The Lancet,* (April 21), 890-894.

Korte, A. O., & Villa, R. F. (1988). Life satisfaction among Hispanic elderly. In M. Sotomayor, & H. Curiel (Eds.), *Hispanic Elderly: A Cultural Signature* (pp. 65-94). Edinburg: Pan American University Press.

Kusserow, R. P. (1984). *A Program Inspection on Hospice Care* (1). Department of Health and Human Services.

Leon, M. (1987). *Access to Health Care in the United States: Results of a 1986 Survey* (Special Report Number Two). Robert Wood Johnson Foundation.

Leyhe, D. L., Gartside, F. E., & Proctor, D. (1972). Medi-Cal patient satisfaction in Watts. *Health Services Reports, 87*(April), 351-359.

Lundgren, L. M., & Chen, S. T. (1986). Hospice concept and implementation in the Black community. *Journal of Community Health Nursing, 3*(3), 137-144.

Lynn, J. (1985). Ethics in hospice care. In L. F. Paradis (Ed.), *Hospice Handbook: A Guide for Managers and Planners* (pp. 303-324). Rockville: Aspen Systems Corporation.

MacDonald, D. (1989). Non-admissions: The other side of the hospice story. *The American Journal of Hospice Care, 6*(2) 17-42.

Martin, C. M. (1984, September). *Statement of the American Hospital Association to the Senate Finance Committee's Subcommittee on Health on Coverage of Hospice Care Under Medicare.* Washington, D.C.

McDonald, R. (1990, 2). Caring enough to reach out: A hospice considers its minority services. *Hospice,* pp. 12-15.

McDonnell, A. (1987). *Quality Hospice Care: Administration, Organization, and Models.* Owings Mills: National Health Publishing.

Meyers, Hal (1990). Where are the minorities? *American Journal of Palliative and Hospice Care, 7*(5), 19.

Mitchell, J., & Register, J. (1984). An exploration of family interaction with the elderly by race, socioeconomic status and residence. *The Gerontologist, 24*(1), 48-54.

Mor, V. (1987a). *Hospice Care Systems: Structure, Process, Costs, and Outcome.* New York: Springer Press.

Mor, V., Greer, D.S., & Kastenbaum, R. (Eds.) (1988). *The Hospice Experiment.* Baltimore: The John Hopkins University Press.

Mor, V., Hendershot, G., & Cryan, C. (1989). Awareness of hospice services: Results of a national survey. *Public Health Reports, 104*(2), 178-182.

Morrow-Howell, N., Lott, L., & Ozawa, M. (1990). The impact of race on volunteer helping relationships among the elderly. *Social Work, 35*(5), 395-402.

Mutran, E. (1985). Intergenerational family support among blacks and whites:

Response to culture or to socioeconomic differences? *Journal of Gerontology,* *40*(3), 382-389.

Neubauer, B. J., & Hamilton, C. L. (1990). Racial differences in attitudes toward hospice care. *The Hospice Journal, 6*(1), 37-48.

Nobles, W. (1974). Africanity: Its role in Black families. *The Black Scholar,* (June), 10-16.

Paradis, L. F. (1984). Hospice: The first DRG. *Health Matrix, II*(4), 32-34.

Pawling-Kaplan, M., & O'Connor, P. (1987). The effect of Medicare on access to hospice care. *The American Journal of Hospice Care, 4*(6), 34-42.

Pawling-Kaplan, M. & O'Connor, P. (1989). Hospice care for minorities: An analysis of a hospital-based inner city palliative care service. *The American Journal of Hospice Care, 6*(4), 13-21.

Rhymes, J. (1990). Hospice care in America. *Journal of the American Medical Association, 264*(3), 369-372.

Richman, J. M., & Rosenfeld, L. B. (1988). Demographic profile of individuals with knowledge of the hospice concept. *The American Journal of Hospice Care, 5*(1), 36-39.

Riessman, C. K. (1986). Improving the health experiences of low income patients. In P. Conrad, & R. Kern (Eds.), *The Sociology of Health and Illness: Critical Perspectives* (pp. 419-432). New York: St. Martin's Press.

Rubel, A. J. (1960). Concepts of disease in Mexican-American culture. *American Anthropologist, 62*(October), 795-814.

Rubenstein, D. (1971). An examination of social participation found among a national sample of Black and White elderly. *Aging and Human Development.* *2*, 172-182.

Sidel, V. W. & Sidel, R. (1983). *A Healthy State: An International Perspective on the Crisis in United States Medical Care* (Second Edition). New York: Pantheon Books.

Solis, J. M., Marks, G., Garcia, M., & Shelton, D. (1990). Acculturation: Access to care, and use of preventive services by Hispanics: Findings from HHANES 1982-84. *American Journal of Public Health, 80*(Supplement), 11-19.

Sotomayor, M. (1988). The Hispanic elderly: A cultural signature. In M. Sotomayor, & H. Curiel (Eds.), *Hispanic Elderly: A Cultural Signature* (pp. 1-10). Edinburg: Pan American University Press.

Sotomayor, M., & Randolph, S. (1988a). The health status of the Hispanic elderly. In M. Sotomayor, & H. Curiel (Eds.), *Hispanic Elderly: A Cultural Signature* (pp. 203-226). Edinburg: Pan American University Press.

Sotomayor, M., & Randolph, S. (1988b). A preliminary review of caregiving issues among Hispanic elderly. In M. Sotomayor, & H. Curiel (Eds.), *Hispanic Elderly: A Cultural Signature* (pp. 137-161). Edinburg: Pan American University Press.

Strauss, A. (1972). Medical ghettos. In E. G. Jaco (Ed.), *Patients, Physicians and Illness* (pp. 381-388). New York: Free Press.

Strauss, A., & Corbin, J. M. (1988). *Shaping a New Health Care System.* San Francisco: Jossey-Bass Inc.

Taylor, R. (1986). The extended family as a source of support to elderly blacks. *The Gerontologist, 25*(5), 488-495.

Taylor, R., & Chatters, L. (1986). Patterns of informal support to elderly black adults. *Social Work, 31*(4), 432-438.

Terrell, F., & Terrell, S. (1981). An inventory to measure cultural mistrust among blacks. *The Western Journal of Black Studies, 5*(3), 180-185.

Torrens, P. R. (1985). Which dying patients should hospices serve? In P. R. Torrens (Ed.), *Hospice Programs and Public Policy* (pp. 63-72). Chicago: American Hospital Publishing, Inc.

U.S. Bureau of the Census (1987). *Statistical Abstract of the United States.* (107th ed.) Washington, D.C.: U.S. Government Printing Office.

Weaver, J. L. (1976). *National Health Policy and the Underserved.* St. Louis: The C. V. Mosby Company.

Identifying and Meeting Needs
of Ethnic Minority Patients

Barbara J. Noggle

SUMMARY. In an effort to meet the unique needs of terminally ill patients and their loved ones within underserved minority populations, hospices are attempting to learn more about the diverse cultures represented in their communities. This paper will discuss one hospice's experience and perceptions of barriers to providing hospice care to individuals of diverse cultural backgrounds and the steps taken to more effectively serve them. *[Single or multiple copies of this article are available from The Haworth Document Delivery Service: 1-800-342-9678, 9:00 a.m. - 5:00 p.m. (EST).]*

INTRODUCTION

What barriers do minority patients experience in accessing hospice care? We have come to a time in the development of this health care service when hospices are compelled to explore the needs of patient populations who fall outside of the mainstream, white, middle-class patients who have been the predominant recipients of hospice care in the United States–patient populations such as children, people with AIDS, non-cancer patients, residents of nursing homes or other facilities, and ethnic minorities.

One by one the barriers excluding these non-traditional hospice popula-

---

Barbara J. Noggle, BSN, is Executive Director, Hospice of the Valley, San Jose, CA.

Address correspondence to: Barbara J. Noggle, Executive Director, Hospice of the Valley, 1150 S. Bascom Avenue, San Jose, CA 95128.

[Haworth co-indexing entry note]: "Identifying and Meeting Needs of Ethnic Minority Patients." Noggle, Barbara J. Co-published simultaneously in *The Hospice Journal* (The Haworth Press, Inc.) Vol. 10, No. 2, 1995, pp. 85-93; and: *Hospice Care and Cultural Diversity* (ed: Donna Lind Infeld, Audrey K. Gordon, and Bernice Catherine Harper) The Haworth Press, Inc., 1995, pp. 85-93. Single or multiple copies of this article are available from The Haworth Document Delivery Service: [1-800-342-9678, 9:00 a.m. - 5:00 p.m. (EST)].

85

tions are falling. Hospice organizations are offering programs on pediatric hospice care, care for people with AIDS and other non-cancer diagnoses, delivering hospice services to people who cannot remain in their own homes, and more recently, on how to make hospice care a fitting option for ethnic minorities.

The place to begin is the same place that was obvious to hospices starting up in the late 1970s: there are people dying who are not receiving hospice care. *We want to serve them.* Therefore, we must learn about these potential patients and their families–their beliefs and hopes, their support systems, their physical, emotional, spiritual and financial needs–and then we must set out to shape our services to fit those needs.

Although the experiences and perceptions described here are based on a hospice in a large metropolitan area in northern California, they are intended to be generalizable and broadly relevant to the experience of hospice caregivers everywhere.

HOSPICE OF THE VALLEY

California leads the nation in the number of new immigrants. Since 1984 the largest number of arrivals in California, in the order of percentage of the total population, have been Mexican, Filipino, Vietnamese, Korean, Asian Indian, and Chinese. Census officials predict that 64 per cent of all new Asians arriving in the United States will live or have already settled in California (Hospice of the Valley, 1988).

Hospice of the Valley (HOV), founded in Santa Clara County in 1979, has experienced a modest, steady census growth of 10 percent per year. Since 1985 HOV's patient population has begun to reflect the county's ethnic population distribution. In five years, the number of Caucasian patients dropped 20 percent while Latino and Asian/Pacific Islander patients increased by 9 percent each. During the same period there has been a 2 percent increase in African American patients while First Americans represent an unchanged 1 percent of yearly census. Figure 1 compares the ethnic diversity of the HOV patient population to Santa Clara County demographics (At work in Silicon Valley, 1993). This gradual shift in HOV's patient demographics between 1985 and 1991/92 can be attributed to two primary factors: (1) Hospice care is often available when no other care is, and (2) an organized HOV outreach effort.

ECONOMIC FACTORS

In the first half of 1992, 20 to 40 percent of HOV's patients had limited or no health insurance coverage. Hospital discharge planners see hospices,

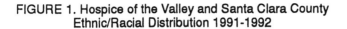

FIGURE 1. Hospice of the Valley and Santa Clara County
Ethnic/Racial Distribution 1991-1992

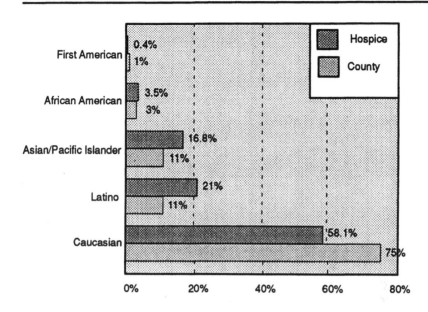

especially those which accept patients without a payment source, as safe havens. Patients and families often do not know what hospice means. Even if they do understand that they are taking their loved one home to care for until death, they may comply because that is their only option. According to the California Health and Safety Code, 60 percent of HOV's total patient census can be defined as low income. While ethnic minorities are no more likely to be in poverty than Caucasians, more patients of all ethnic groups may be coming into hospice care because it is available when other care is not.

OVERCOMING BARRIERS TO SERVING ETHNIC MINORITIES

In 1988, recognizing the need to expand hospice services to ethnic minorities, HOV engaged a volunteer to survey 11 minority groups in the county (See Appendix). She identified minority community leaders, members of social service organizations serving minority clients, and representatives from the County Health Department. A questionnaire elicited attitudes about traditions, rituals and beliefs surrounding terminal illness, accepting help from "outsiders," treatments and medical interventions, and death and after-death. Follow-up personal interviews clarified and amplified responses.

The material was then compiled into a handbook, *Ethnic Diversity and the Care of the Terminally Ill in Santa Clara County,* designed as a guide for hospice workers. The handbook was distributed to interdisciplinary team members and to be used as a reference. The County Medical Society became aware of the Handbook and asked permission to reprint and distribute 315 copies, without charge, to physicians, nursing facilities, and hospitals.

The introduction to the handbook acknowledges that each individual and family within any ethnic group is indeed unique. The material encourages each hospice worker to move out from behind the frame of his or her particular perspective to explore how previously-considered universal principles of care may be tinged with personal or cultural values and assumptions. Further, it describes how the normative American view of the meaning of health and illness is not the same as that of other ethnic and national groups.

While patients subscribe to cultural standards to varying degrees, the extent to which they adhere to ethnic standards of health behavior is related to their acculturation to American norms. However, even patients who generally display low adherence to ethnic culture may resort to ethnically-derived, nonmainstream modes of health behavior in certain situations, especially those involving great emotional stress, such as terminal illness (Harwood, 1981).

It was the experience of HOV that hospice workers open their personal windows when provided information about other cultural practices and beliefs. Values and assumptions change and new understanding leads to appreciation. Demystification is evidenced when a hospice worker becomes so comfortable and accepting of another culture that significant differences are not even noted in day-to-day patient encounters. For example, one nurse interviewed for this study said, "When I was asked about the ethnic minority families I have served, I couldn't think of any." She went on, "I have done my most miraculous stuff with cultures I know nothing about. If you don't know anything about a culture, you are not tempted to come up with your own solutions for them." This response reflects the ideal attributes of a hospice worker: accepting, supportive, and non-interfering. Another hospice nurse, an African American, observed, "For a black hospice nurse, ethnic clarity no longer is a primary issue–the experience of dying is the primary issue. Just like when everyone is in an earthquake together, everyone looks the same."

Heartwarming and reassuring as these two nurses' perceptions are, there remain real barriers to cross-cultural caregiving. Language is one. A respite volunteer stated, "You don't need to have a common language for what we do, at the point we do it. Eighty percent of language is body language." However, making oneself understood when explaining a medication regimen, fielding a crisis over the telephone, or obtaining reliable information to develop a plan of care, can be ineffective, frustrating, or even dangerous when one individual cannot understand the other. Few hospices have staff available to interpret in every language, especially during on-call hours.

Family members, typically the younger generation, may become interpreters. However, they may tend to "screen" information in an attempt to protect the patient's dignity, feelings, or imagined point of view. Churches or clubs may be able to supply volunteer interpreters. This task is critical as hospice work calls for understanding of denotative (what words stand for) and connotative (what words suggest) aspects of the language which used to describe symptoms (Thernstrom, 1980).

Hospice is about offering choices to patients and their families. Language barriers severely limit one's understanding of available choices. For example, patients have the right to receive maximum comfort measures, but if a nurse is not able to make herself understood when explaining how to increase the effectiveness of pain medication, the patient has lost some level of choice and control.

For minority families, hospice care may be seen as intruding, with activities of hospice workers in direct conflict with cultural norms. For example, with great courtesy the Asian family may say "thank you" over and over again and would really rather a caregiver was not there at all.

Communication failure can lead to lack of trust. New immigrants are forced to become part of a medical bureaucracy they often do not understand. They may believe the medical profession is experimenting on them, especially if their care is paid for by a government program. They may mistrust the doctor's diagnosis and wonder if they are receiving the same care as other patients. They question their value in the eyes of the medical profession.

Even if language is not an issue, belonging to a minority culture may result in feelings of discrimination or inequality. Discrimination may be a new experience for recent immigrants who may have not been members of a cultural minority in their home country. Hospices are just one more arm of the health care and social work system, telling them what to do and snooping in their business. When hospice patients and their families feel inferior, they may appear compliant for fear that providers will walk out on them.

On the other hand, immigrant patients may think hospice caregivers will take over and try to change things. They may have very little experience with people not of their own culture being caring and supportive members of their lives. They have many business contacts (stores, social service agencies, gas stations), but few caring contacts. As with all other families, trust remains the touchstone for dealing with dying patients and their loved ones. Trust and thoughtfulness were the two most important aspects of caring for dying patients noted by people of all races and national origins surveyed for the HOV Handbook (Hospice of the Valley, 1988).

COMMUNITY EDUCATION AND PUBLIC RESPONSES

According to Chai (1987), "there are about 100 identifiable ethnic groups in the United States . . . sometimes, maybe too often, health care providers view and treat these groups as homogeneous. We fail to recognize that the subcultures within each ethnic group differ and reflect a unique set of socio-historical forces." This observation bears heavily on a hospice's community outreach plan. Who do we talk to? How do we talk to them? What human and financial resources are available to publish information and provide speakers to address the full population of the service area about the availability and benefits of hospice care?

HOV has published information in Spanish, explaining the goals of hospice care, symptom management, and what to do as death approaches. Working with a hospice volunteer for whom Spanish was a second language, the content was designed to accurately reflect hospice services. Following broad distribution among the Spanish-speaking community, to our chagrin, an elderly Mexican-American woman said that, to her, "hospicio" meant a place for indigents. The whole idea of hospice care was thus clouded by miscommunication. Each language contains nuances which may create barriers to understanding. Therefore, it is imperative that translators understand, with some depth, the technology and the spirit of hospice care; Literal translations will miss the mark. As we strive to get the message out, we must check and double check that what we *say* in another language is what we *mean*. HOV has now also published materials in Vietnamese. One by one, the other languages spoken in our community will also receive translations.

The ethnic press and radio has also been of considerable influence. While their need to popularize information may lead to potential distortions, hospice providers should consider these channels in disseminating information to people of all class and ethnic backgrounds (Harwood, 1981). Translators who know hospice and know the culture of the people they are educating, not just the language, are most likely to accurately convey the hospice message. It is, therefore, important to recruit and train individuals for hospice speakers' bureaus who are members of the cultures the hospice is trying to reach.

Hospice of the Valley, in cooperation with other local agencies, is currently planning a community-wide forum directed at an audience of nurses, doctors, social workers, and other health care providers. Minority panelists will be drawn from local universities and other organizations. A discussion of cultural attitudes and taboos related to health care is designed to foster greater understanding and sensitivity on the part of all providers.

Finally, recruiting minority volunteers, at every level, such as board members and respite and bereavement workers, poses an important and worthwhile challenge. HOV has had limited success in attracting and retaining volunteers who reflect the diverse cultural mix of its patient population. Many potentially volunteers work several jobs and are therefore not available. In addition, for many minorities, volunteerism is not a cultural norm and therefore has no personal or group value. It simply is not done. So while hospices work diligently to develop community outreach and promote understanding they lack assistance from those who could have the greatest effect.

CONCLUSION

Certain challenges arise for hospices attempting to identify and respond to the needs of ethnic minority patients. Many of the considerations are the same when hospice care is provided to any other patient, but others are culturally specific. Although language differences and unfamiliar beliefs and cultural practices create barriers, they can be overcome. Hospice caregivers need to be offered the opportunity to learn about cultural diversity, enabling them to give the best possible care. Meeting these challenges calls on hospice workers' most important attributes–being open, non-judgmental, sensitive, and willing to learn.

REFERENCES

Population by ethnicity in Santa Clara County (graph) (1993). At work in the Silicon Valley. *The Business Journal* (Supplement), May, 10.
Chai, M. (1987). Older Asians. *Journal of gerontological nursing*, (3)11; 11.
Cohen, Lucy M. (1979). *Culture, Disease, and Stress Among Latino Immigrants*, Washington, D.C.: Smithsonian Institution.

Harwood, Alan (Ed.) (1981). *Ethnicity and Medical Care*, Cambridge, MA: Harvard University Press.
Hospice of the Valley (1988). *Ethnic Diversity and the Care of the Terminally Ill in Santa Clara County: A Handbook*, San Jose, CA.
Thernstrom, Stephan (1980) *Harvard encyclopedia of American ethnic groups*. Cambridge, MA: Belknap Press.

APPENDIX

HOV ETHNIC COMMUNITY RESEARCH SURVEY

Name of organization: _____

Address: _____

Phone number: _____

Contact name: _____

Ethnic community: _____

1. DEMOGRAPHIC INFORMATION

    A. Estimated population in Santa Clara County _____

    B. Location of population centers within the city.

    C. Key community organizations and/or individuals (list names, contacts, and phone numbers).

    D. Community newspaper, radio stations, cable TV, publications (list names, contacts, and phone numbers).

    E. Religious organizations (list names, contacts, and phone numbers).

    F. Medical community (list names and phone numbers for Physicians, Clinics/Health Centers, and professional organizations (nurses, doctors, social workers).

    G. Translation services (names, contacts, phone numbers).

    H. Support services (organized or informal) that relate to in-home care for very ill/dying people (names, contacts, phone numbers, and service descriptions).

2. CULTURAL ATTITUDES REGARDING:

Death
Dying at home
Family as caregivers
Non-family members as caregivers
Gender of caregiver(s)
Pain medications
Medical assistance/alternative healing approaches
English words about death/dying with negative connotations
Volunteerism/community involvement
Other issues/cultural attitudes to which we should be sensitive

3. SUGGESTIONS FOR CONTINUED OUTREACH:

Speaking opportunities (i.e., churches, civic groups. Programs available from 10 minutes to 2 hours. Can include film video).

Printed literature (e.g., Spanish and Vietnamese brochures)

Volunteer recruitment (review volunteer opportunities)

Other suggestions for outreach

4. WOULD YOU LIKE TO BE PLACED ON OUR MAILING LIST?

Interview conducted by: _____

Date:_____   Phone: _____

Index

Activities of daily living (ADLs)
    limitations, of Hispanic-
    American elders, 36
Acculturation continuum, 38
African Americans
    attitudes towards death and dying,
        71-72,73,74
    hospice care access, barriers to,
        15-18
        cultural barriers, 73-74
        lack of trust in hospice
            caregivers, 73-74
    lack of medical care for, 70
    life expectancy of, 72
    physician visits by, 20
Animistic folk beliefs, of Cambodians,
    55,57-58
Anxiety, of Cambodian refugees, 61
AT&T Language Line, 5

Beckwith, Samira K., 5
Bereavement, among children
    of Cambodian children
        bereavement programs for,
            61-62
        caregiver availability during,
            60-61
        cultural beliefs affecting,
            58-59
        educational factors affecting,
            59-60
        effect of post-traumatic stress
            disorder on, 53,55
        obstacles to, 59-61
        recommendations for, 61-62
        religious beliefs affecting,
            55-58
    caregiver availability during,
        54-55,60-61

children's communication of grief
    during, 54
environmental stability during,
    54-55
of Israeli children, 54
Billingsley, Sydney, 5
Brahmanism, 55
Brown University, National Hospice
    Study, 2
Buddhism
    beliefs about death and dying,
        55,56-57
    Khmer, 55
    Theravada, 55,57-58

California Health and Safety Code, 87
Cambodian children, grief resolution by
    bereavement programs for, 61-62
    caregiver availability during,
        60-61
    cultural beliefs affecting, 58-59
    educational factors affecting,
        59-60
    effect of post-traumatic stress
        disorder on, 53,54
    obstacles to, 59-61
    recommendations for, 61-62
    religious beliefs affecting, 55-58
Cancer, incidence among African-
    Americans, 72
Caregivers
    African-American, 17,74,75-
        76,78
    for bereaved children, 54-55,
        60-61
    Hispanic-American, 37-38,40
        case examples of, 42-45
        depression in, 37
    Mexican-American, 75

Printed and bound by CPI Group (UK) Ltd, Croydon, CR0 4YY

22/10/2024

01777615-0010